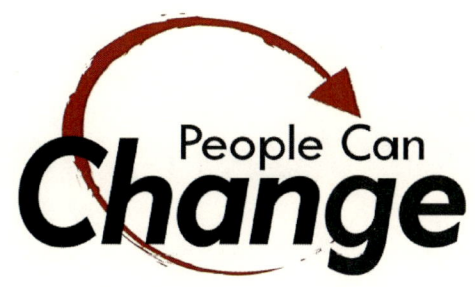

# Then & Now:

## How My Sexual Attractions Have Changed

### 50 Brief Summaries of Successful

### Sexual Orientation Change Efforts

Overview chapters by Rich Wyler,
Founder and Executive Director of People Can Change, Inc.

First-person accounts compiled and edited by Rich Wyler
Cover design by Stephen Jacobs

Published by People Can Change, Inc., Virginia USA

# About People Can Change

<u>People Can Change</u> is a non-profit educational, support and outreach organization founded in 2000 in Virginia, USA. It is best known for its life-changing <u>Journey Into Manhood</u> weekend experience, which People Can Change offers across the U.S. and in Europe and Israel. People Can Change is not a religious ministry and is not affiliated with any religious faith or organization.

- **Our Mission:** "To support and guide men who seek to transition away from unwanted homosexuality, by courageously and compassionately sharing our own first-hand experience with change. We also provide information and support to friends and family, especially wives."

- **Our Vision:** "We envision a world in which all people with unwanted same-sex attractions who wish to reduce or eliminate their homosexual feelings have access to meaningful and effective resources and successful role models, and are free to pursue a path of change, if they so choose, without shame or ridicule."

# What Do We Mean By "Change"?

An excerpt from <u>www.peoplecanchange.com</u>:

Some skeptics erroneously assume that by "change" we always mean (or *should* mean) a 180 degree shift from 100% homosexual to 100% heterosexual in all behaviors, interests, attractions and thoughts, forever after. Anything less than that, some critics argue, isn't real change. Some look for evidence of "only" a 170 degree shift or "only" a 90 degree shift, and cry "failure!"

The truth is that any degree of change toward greater peace, satisfaction and fulfillment, and less shame, depression and darkness, is change well worth pursuing.

For most people who seek change, heterosexuality is not actually the ultimate goal—happiness and peace are.

And for us, happiness and peace are not contingent on sexuality alone, but on living a life congruent with our deeply held values, beliefs and life goals.

So, unlike those who argue that nothing less than a 180 degree turn "counts" as change, those of us who actually experience change are often quite content with a much subtler shift.

- To be free from the constant pull of homosexual desires.

- To have deeply fulfilling non-sexual friendships with other men, and to belong to a close community of men.

- Perhaps to have a happy marriage, to be a loving father, or else to be contentedly single.

- To live a life we feel is aligned with God's will for us.

Many of us could ask for nothing more.[1]

---

[1]   http://www.peoplecanchange.com/change/whatwemean.php

# Table of Contents

# Why This Book?

Over the past decade or two, it has become "common knowledge" that homosexuality is inborn, innate, and unchangeable—that, in fact, any attempt to change one's sexual orientation will inevitably cause great psychological harm and perhaps even lead to suicide.

Everybody knows that, right?

Wrong.

In fact, this "common knowledge" isn't science; it's ideology. These aren't facts; they are talking points. But through relentless repetition, these ideas have entered the mainstream consciousness until it appears to be one of those things that simply "everyone knows" to be true. (There is a saying widely known among those who are professionally engaged in attempting to sway public opinion: "People will believe a big lie sooner than a little one, and if you repeat it frequently enough, people will sooner or later believe it."[2])

Our own experience is quite different. We *know* change in sexual attractions is possible—at least to some degree, and at least for some people—because we've experienced it ourselves. No appeal to position papers, talking points, "expert" opinion or even research studies can disprove our own lived experience. We know it because we've lived it.

By telling you we've experienced change—and that we are better and happier for it—we are *not* saying that *everyone* can change, or *anyone* can change, or everyone *should* change (or try to). We are *not* saying that being gay is bad or wrong for everyone or a mental disorder or mental defect or even sinful. We are *not* saying that gays can't find love, that they are unhappy or inevitably will be unhappy, or that they should have any fewer civil rights protections or be treated differently by the law than anyone else.

No, all we are saying is that homosexuality was wrong *for us*, so we pursued a path of sexual-orientation change. This path worked *for us*, and brought us greater peace, brotherhood, and self-esteem than we had ever known before. So we can only assume that similar efforts may work for some others as well, if they are dissatisfied with or conflicted about their same-sex attractions and want to explore the possibility of change.

That's why we've compiled this book: to share our own experience with others who might benefit—others who are now where we ourselves were not that long ago.

This is the first edition of a growing collection of first-hand accounts of men who successfully engaged in sexual-orientation change efforts, collected and compiled (and lightly edited for space, clarity, punctuation and grammar) by People Can Change.

## About the Questionnaire

How did People Can Change gather these stories into this publication?

In late 2013, we sent out a questionnaire to our online data base of past and potential participants in our programs. The email requested "personal accounts demonstrating that, yes, some people really have reduced or eliminated their same-sex attractions through deliberate interventions like counseling, experiential weekend programs, non-sexual same-gender bonding, etc."

---

[2] Psychoanalyst Walter Langer

A total of 178 people responded to all or portions of the questionnaire. Almost all of them were men, since this is the significant majority of the population that People Can Change serves (along with wives of men who deal with unwanted same-sex attractions or sex addictions). From these 178 responses, People Can Change has culled a diverse sampling of 50 (well, 54, actually) personal accounts of sexual-orientation change efforts, which we share with you here. Future editions of this book will include even more.

Among all those who responded to the PCC questions:

- 83% reported a complete, major or moderate reduction in their same-sex attractions.
- 59% reported a complete, major or moderate transition to opposite-sex attractions.

Others reported a less dramatic shift (or none at all) in their sexual attractions, but still noted how much they had benefited from their sexual-orientation change efforts (abbreviated "SOCE").

## Anecdotal and Qualitative

Neither the original 178 questionnaire responses nor these 50-plus first-hand accounts constitute an unbiased or representative sampling of all those who have ever engaged in sexual-orientation change efforts. This is not quantitative research. There are no statistical projections that can be drawn from this sampling of first-hand accounts.

In developing this book, we were specifically looking for success stories. We sent the questionnaire to our own data base of participants and prospective participants—so we were far more likely to find success stories than to find people dissatisfied with their change efforts.

The value of these accounts is in what we can learn from the responses about what worked, which resources were most helpful—and most especially, the reality of change (however individuals may define "change" for themselves). The questionnaire and this book cannot tell you how often change occurs, or how likely change is to occur. But they do demonstrate that, yes, change *does in fact occur*. It's real. It can even be life-saving.

These accounts also demonstrate what "change" means for different people. They show that someone doesn't have to experience a 180-degree shift in sexual attractions to experience a profound increase in peace, love and growth. The goal of most sexual-orientation change efforts is not really heterosexuality, after all. It is peace.

## "SSA" and "OSA"

Gay communities have embraced the term "gay" since at least the 1960s over the more clinically sounding or sexually charged word "homosexual," and the world has largely respected their preference and followed suit. However, men and women who feel sexually attracted to others of the same sex *but who resist or even seek to change those attractions* typically don't embrace the identity of "gay." To us, the word is too politically loaded, too indicative of a "gay pride" that we don't feel and refuse to embrace, and too aligned with gay liberal ideologies with which we often disagree.

Since at least the 1980s, psychologists have referred to this state of mind as "ego-dystonic homosexuality," referring to those who experience cognitive and emotional dissonance over their homosexual attractions. Talk about sounding clinical! Then, in the 1991 book, Reparative Therapy of Male Homosexuality, author and psychologist Joseph Nicolosi introduced the term "non-gay homosexual." It never caught on.

Among ourselves, the preferred term is usually "same-sex attracted," or SSA. It suggests a present condition or state, not a permanent identity. It implies a feeling, not a sense of self. SSA is "what I feel, not who I am." It doesn't align us with what we find so off-putting about gay lifestyles and gay politics. Nor does it have the overly clinical or sexualized ring that the term "homosexual" has.

In fact, the phrase "same-sex attracted" and its acronym SSA have been widely embraced throughout the world by men and women who decline to let their sexual attractions define them or to identify with the politics and ideologies of gay cultures.

Also, as a simple matter of shorthand (and equivalency?), SSA men and women may in turn sometimes refer to heterosexuality as "opposite-sex attraction," or OSA. This term hasn't caught on nearly as widely, however.

And what about the term "ex-gay"? It's convenient shorthand, perhaps, but that may be about the extent of its virtue. Most SSA men and women don't use it, or don't identify with it, although they usually aren't offended by it either. Most SSA men and women had simply never embraced a gay identity to begin with, so how can they embrace an "ex-gay" identity now?

In truth, most of us don't care much for labeling our sexuality. It's often too complex, too nuanced for a convenient label, and we would simply rather not reduce ourselves to an abbreviation or to a politicized term. But the demands of human communication today often require the use of sound-bite terms that convey shared meaning succinctly. So in our communities, we typically choose to call ourselves "SSA" or someone "dealing with unwanted SSA" or similar phrasing, rather than "gay." Or, if it fits better, we may refer to ourselves as "formerly SSA" or someone "from an SSA background."

That's our prerogative. We get to decide. Gay communities—just because they are vastly larger in numbers and louder in their demands—don't get to dictate how we refer to ourselves.

## Real Names and Pseudonyms

The People Can Change questionnaire asked respondents if PCC could use their real name (first name only) in relating their personal stories. Almost half said yes and half said no.

- In this book, real first names are given without quotation marks, like this: Jeremy.

- Aliases are written within quotation marks, like this: "Rob."

But you may ask the question: Why are so many of these men unwilling to provide their real names?

For some, it is out of fear of retribution. Those who have been public with their experience know the sting of being mocked and maligned for daring to speak out against the "gay party line" (born that way, can't change, change efforts are always harmful, etc.). Some have had their employment threatened and even received death threats.

For some, it is a desire to put the past in the past. Most SSA men were never publicly gay, so being "formerly gay" is not an identity they want to publicly embrace. They don't want their sexual histories to define them.

For everyone, there is careful consideration for personal "reputation management," particularly in today's social-media-drenched world where anything can become part of the online public record for a lifetime.

Regardless of whether these men choose to use their real first name or an alias, they show a great deal of courage by sharing their stories here. They do it out of concern for others who are now where we once were.

## Why Just Men?

Why does this book focus just on men? Simply because that's who we at People Can Change primarily serve. Our programs are designed for men with unwanted SSA, as well as their wives, if they are married. So it's the men whose stories we know and whose contact information we have. That's who we are able to reach out to in order to ask them to share their success stories.

# Our Lives "Then"

We've called this book "Then & Now" because in it we give a snapshot of our lives before we began our sexual-orientation change efforts and compare that to our lives now. Sort of a "before and after" picture, if you will. Of course, you can't exactly take a snapshot of sexual-orientation change. It's a lot harder to demonstrate than weight loss or muscle gain like we see in the infomercials. Sexual-orientation change is much subtler, more nuanced, and not measurable by mere observation. All we can do is share our own lived experience, then and now.

The questionnaire sent out by People Can Change asked: ***At the time when your same-sex attraction (SSA) was the most intense, how would you have rated the degree of same-sex versus opposite-sex attractions?***

People Can Change asked respondents to indicate one of seven possible options on a range from "exclusively homosexual" to "exclusivel y heterosexual." This is essentially what's known as a Kinsey Scale, or a Heterosexual-Homosexual Rating Scale, developed by psychologist Alfred Kinsey in the 1940s. In their responses, more than three-quarters of respondents described themselves as either "exclusively homosexual" or "primarily homosexual, but with incidental heterosexual attractions" at the point in their lives when the SSA was most intense.

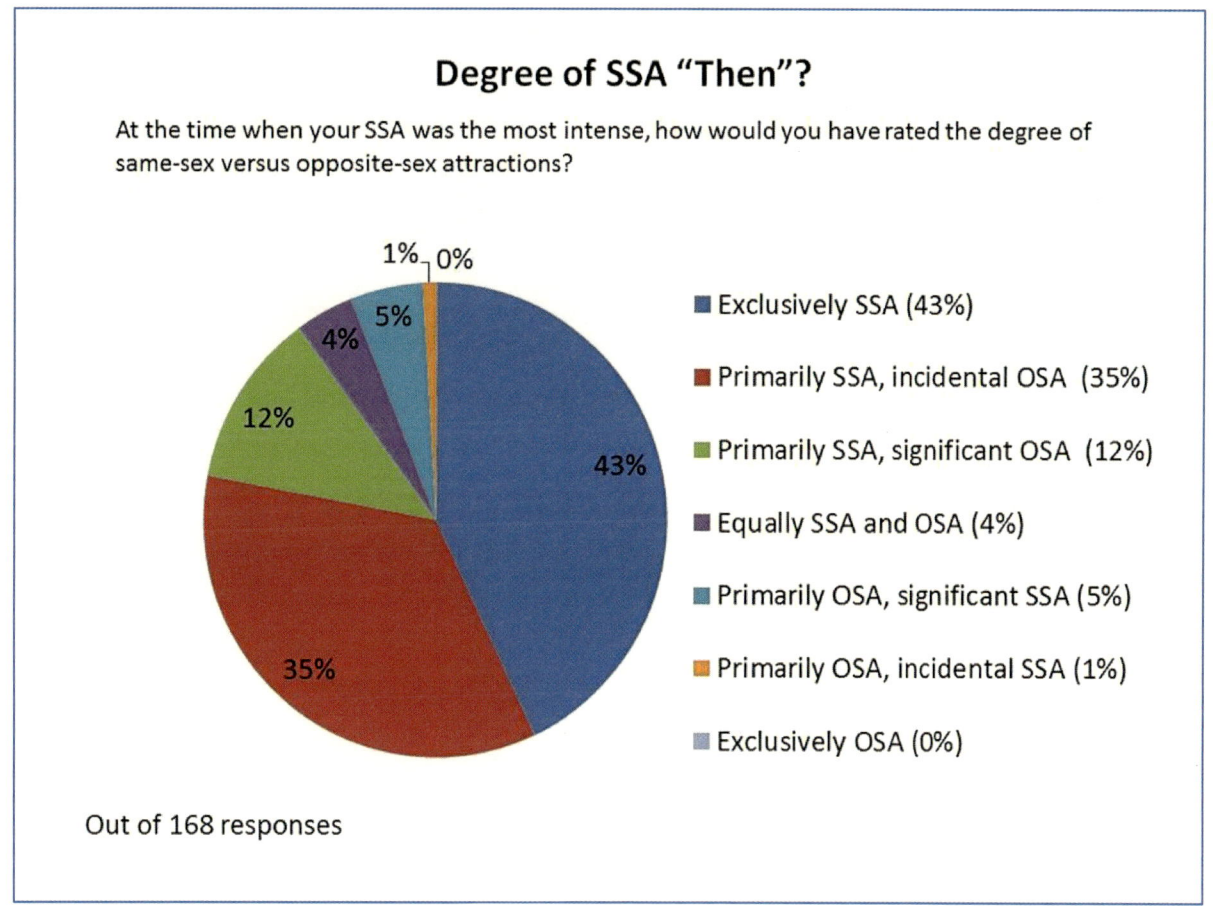

**Degree of SSA "Then"?**

At the time when your SSA was the most intense, how would you have rated the degree of same-sex versus opposite-sex attractions?

- Exclusively SSA (43%)
- Primarily SSA, incidental OSA (35%)
- Primarily SSA, significant OSA (12%)
- Equally SSA and OSA (4%)
- Primarily OSA, significant SSA (5%)
- Primarily OSA, incidental SSA (1%)
- Exclusively OSA (0%)

Out of 168 responses

*The pie charts in this book present a <u>profile</u> of those who responded to the People Can Change questionnaire from which the 54 brief summaries were drawn. They do not indicate representative samplings of SSA or gay populations or of all those who have attempted sexual-orientation changes.*

Also, based on responses to open-ended questions, it appears that:

- About 10% of the men who answered the questions had been openly gay at one time, including previously being in long-term gay relationships.

- Between a quarter and a third of all respondents had never acted on their same-sex attractions with other men (although many had been heavily involved in pornography and homosexual fantasy).

- About six in 10 respondents had "acted out" secretly in the past, had had secret affairs, or had lived a secret "double life" of an outwardly heterosexual man (sometimes married) and a closeted gay man.

More significantly, though, is the quality of life the respondents described at the time in their lives when their SSA was most intense. The questionnaire asked:

***Please share briefly about your experience with same-sex attraction before you made any meaningful change effort. As a reference point, you might think about a time in your life when the SSA seemed the strongest, or when you were most conflicted, or when it was most challenging for you.***

The responses are striking. We share them here, not to suggest that these are necessarily common experiences for gay men generally. But they do seem to be common experiences for men who experience *unwanted* same-sex attraction, or who are deeply conflicted about their same-sex attractions over a long period of time. These responses reveal a lot about the "SSA experience"—and a lot about the kinds of things that can motive men like us to pursue change.

(For more, see responses in the "SSA Then" row of each of the 54 brief summaries.)

# Inner Turmoil

Many men in the questionnaire shared about the great inner turmoil and conflict they experienced at that time of their lives, and how miserable they felt. For example:

- "Prior to seeking help, I was in agonizing turmoil. …The inner conflict became so severe that I was often suicidal—and attempted once."

— Kevin, 29, Idaho, page 49

- "I thought that if I just accepted the reality that I was gay, my 'acting out' would decrease. However, I found that identifying as gay did not sit well with who I really felt I was inside. I was in constant turmoil, living a lie no matter which way I turned."

— Carmine, 69, Indiana, page 95

- "I was depressed, compulsive, angry, hyper-sexual and avoidant. I was closeted and shamed. I was suicidal. I was outed and shamed more. I wanted to die."

— "Monty," 24, New York, page 86

- "I never came out publicly, but I did my best to embrace the [gay] lifestyle. ... I was very conflicted, and came to the point of being suicidal. I was very unhappy and started using drugs and alcohol to try to feel better. This only made it worse."

— Robert, 47, Texas, page 76

- "I was a self-affirmed, out-of-the-closet, fully identified gay man. I was in a relationship with another man for 18 years. I had absolutely no heterosexual desire. By the world's standards, I was moderately successful. We owned a house, had two cars and many friends. Yet deep down inside I was miserable. I was very sexually active with many partners. And I felt completely empty."

— Ronald, 50, California, page 82

# Out-of-Control Sexual Behaviors

Many shared about out-of-control sexual behaviors that directly violated their deeply held morals and values:

- "At my worst, I was hooking up with men as often as four to five times a week, usually different men."

  — Kevin, 40, California, page 70

- "Between 14 and 35, I was sexually addicted to pornography, sex with many different men, and masturbation. I was unhappy with all this: my sexuality, my shame about my own body and manhood, my compulsive desire for the body of other men."

  — Stefan, 41, Germany, page 71

- "I 'acted out' with men secretly. These encounters were mostly in public places and with anonymous men I had never met before. I never even knew their names. ... Over time, the amount of 'acting out' increased and, at times, this behavior would become obsessive and compulsive. ... I was sad, depressed and had difficulty sleeping. I also felt shame and guilt with regard to my behavior. I wanted to stop, but couldn't."

  — Steve, 55, Florida, page 103

- "No matter how much sex I had or how many chat rooms I was in, something just didn't feel right, and I still needed more. I drank more and more and started making a plan to live on the streets as a male prostitute. I figured it would mean I would take street drugs and be dead before age 25—and I was fine with that."

  — Tim, 37, Idaho, page 45

# Loneliness and Detachment

Quite a few respondents expressed a deep sense of loneliness and detachment from other males:

- "At its most challenging point, I felt compelled to have sex with men, not because I wanted to be in a gay relationship, but because I felt inferior and unaccepted by other men. Having sex with men increased my self-esteem temporarily, but left me feeling depressed afterward, because what I really wanted was to feel accepted and loved by men *non-sexually.*"

  — Christopher, 33, Virginia, page 41

- "I lived a double life of a gay man and a prefect son. I was absolutely unhappy. I felt alone and wasn't able to relate to anybody."

  — Stephan, 34, Germany, page 58

- "I felt so detached from my own gender and wanted closeness, recognition and affirmation from an older male."

  — Ali, 25, England, page 42

- "Before I started working on my SSA, I felt alone and isolated. I was addicted to same-sex pornography and I knew that was just the beginning. I identified myself as someone who had SSA, and I didn't think change was possible. I was extremely unhappy with myself and was even suicidal at times."

  — Sam, 26, Utah, page 47

- "I longed for male acceptance and belonging, and porn helped turn that natural longing into lust, then addiction. When I visited places that sold porn, men sought me out and gave me attention and (momentary) affection. I was hooked, but horribly conflicted."

  — Rich, 53, Virginia, page 106

7

With experiences and feelings like this, is it any wonder that men like us would seek out help to minimize or eliminate our same-sex attractions?

Our experience is our own. We do not mean to suggest that our experience is necessarily the typical gay experience. But it was our reality. It was how we experienced unwanted homosexual behaviors and attractions. It was the dark, lonely, self-destructive underside of homosexuality that drove us to pursue freedom.

# Why Pursue Change?

Given the extent of unhappiness and discontent described in these 50-plus first-person accounts, is it any wonder that men like us would attempt to alter or diminish the same-sex attractions that were causing us so much distress?

The <u>People Can Change</u> questionnaire asked, ***"What motivates (or motivated) you to seek to diminish your homosexual attractions or shift toward more heterosexual attractions?"*** Answers tended to fall into about six categories:

1. General disappointment with gay life, gay relationships or gay communities.

2. Deep internal conflict with religious or spiritual convictions and personal belief.

3. A strong desire to have a wife and children, or to maintain an existing marriage and family.

4. A perception that, for many of us, homosexuality was a way to cope with underlying pain or unmet longings.

5. A general sense that "gay" was not a core, authentic identity for many of us, or that homosexuality just felt wrong.

6. General unhappiness with life, or a general desire to find peace and fulfillment, and to be a better man overall.

Following are highlights of these responses. For more, see the "Motivations" row in each of the 54 brief summaries.

## Disappointment with Gay Life

Disappointment with gay life, gay relationships or with our experience in gay communities was a key motivating factor for a number of men. The reality we experienced just didn't match the fantasy or the media portrayals. Some examples:

- "The gay community just didn't meet my needs. I didn't identify with gays."
  —Maurice, 36, Alabama, page 60

- "I eventually came to the conclusion that gay relationships were never going to be fulfilling for me, and I wanted to find another alternative."
  — Jeremy, 36, Texas, page 39

- "When I imagined my best fantasy—I'm out and proud, everyone loves me, and I live happily ever after with the man of my dreams—it somehow felt like a consolation prize."
  —Tim, 37, Idaho, page 45

- "What I saw of the men I knew who had gone into the homosexual lifestyle was unappealing. It seemed to me to be a world of promiscuity, and lacked depth. I was looking for a committed family of men to be in my life, and it seemed to me that I wouldn't necessarily find that level of fidelity in the homosexual community. In addition, I didn't see anyone in an openly gay life who I wanted to be like. I wanted to live life as a man, not defining myself by whatever my sexual impulses may be."
  —Tim, 48, Oregon, page 56

- "Being in the gay life in Manhattan generated a rush of excitement that I initially mistook for self-fulfillment. But the lifestyle and my behavior were still driven by my deep insecurity and emotional neediness. I was easily manipulated, and when the rush of an 'encounter' wore off, I felt lonely and bad about myself. ...Deep dissatisfaction with the gay lifestyle, and a desire to live a physically and emotionally healthier life, motivated me to pursue change."

—"David," 52, Israel, page 50

- "When I have acted on homosexual attractions, it has always left me with a bad feeling afterward."

—Sam, 26, Utah, page 47

- "The gay world (or at least gay Los Angeles in the late 1980s) greatly disappointed me. I found in it an obsession with sex, porn, youth and physical appearance; prevalent recreational drug use; a campy, effeminate 'crush' on masculinity; and derision of family, monogamy and religion. I didn't like the man I became when I was with gay boyfriends or at their parties."

—Rich, 53, Virginia, page 106

# Faith and Belief

Religious or spiritual faith and personal beliefs were strong motivators for a lot of men to resolve their unwanted SSA:

- "My religious beliefs cause me to see that there is something higher than myself, and if I want to be in line with that, then I should live the way that I believe will make me happy. The way to my happiness is through living in line with my personal beliefs, religion, and the lifestyle that I choose."

— Jason, 22, Utah, Latter-day Saint, page 43

- "What motivated me to shift my sexual attraction was my faith. I am an orthodox Jewish man, and I was resigned to the 'fact' that I would never be married or loved by a wife. In spite of being a rational, 'modern' thinker, I won't give up my faith."

—Yeshaya, 23, New York, Jewish, page 40

- "[My primary motivation was] my belief in God and my personal convictions. I knew that I was living a lie and that the only way out was to seek God and then to participate in counseling."

— Samuel, 38, South Africa, Christian (Pentecostal), page 68

- "I wanted to live as the man God had created me to be, at peace with his desires, and at peace with other men and women."

— Stefan, 41, Germany, Catholic, page 71

- "After 18 years of living a gay lifestyle, I had come to an end of myself. I did not like anything about who I was and where I was going. I grew up in a Christian household and decided that I would give God one more chance. I had tried everything else in order to make myself feel better and more connected. Nothing worked. It was in a life of submission to the Lordship of Jesus Christ that I found my answer. He is what motivates me to live the life I live now. I often say that the opposite of homosexuality is not heterosexuality, it is holiness. It is living a life based on biblical principles, honoring God and serving Jesus and other people."

— Ronald, 50, California, Christian, page 82

- "At 21, I realized that my religion was more important than the transient nature of this life, and if God didn't want me to act in a certain way then I accepted His authority over my life."

— Mohamed, 34, United Kingdom, Muslim, page 54

# Wife and Family

A strong desire to have a wife and children of their own—or to hold together the marriage and family they already had—was a significant motivator for many men.

- "I wanted to get married to a woman and to live according to my biological sexuality."

  — "Eli," 60, Israel, page 98

- "I was committed to maintaining my marriage and living in harmony with my personal values."

  — Kevin, 29, Idaho, page 49

- "I desired a life that was more compatible with my personal goals as far as family, marriage, children, etc."

  — David, 41, Arizona, page 72

- "I strongly desire to find my soulmate of the opposite sex and to be a father."

  — Charles, 25, France and Turkey, page 65

# SSA Was Covering Underlying Problems

Some men perceived that, for them, SSA did not represent their authentic, inborn sexuality but was a way to cope with underlying pain or unmet longings:

- "I realized that my homosexual desires were an escape from my self-hatred and shame, from real friendships with other men and their emotions, and from women. I realized that I used sex only to reduce distress and not because of real love and relationships."

  — Stefan, 41, Germany, page 71

- "I knew that underneath my SSA were wounds that I didn't know what to do with. I was sexually abused as a pre-teen… and I could sense that my desire for men increased dramatically after that, mainly because my need for attention and acceptance escalated."

  — Kevin, 40, California, page 70

- "I was motivated to change when I accepted that the roots of my unwanted SSA were not a spiritual issue, but that of a wounded boy who had never had a healthy nurturing fathering, and were profoundly emotional and psychological in nature."

  — Dan, 49, South Carolina, page 79

- "I began to understand that what I was really seeking was non-sexual affirmation from the world of men. Sexual gratification never filled the underlying void. I felt deep in my core that I was not homosexual; rather, I had sexualized those male qualities I judged I never possessed."

  — Chuck, 56, Florida, page 88

- "It became obvious that this lust for older, strong and good-looking men matched the absence of and longing for my father, who died when I was 2 years old. …The loss of my father and the lack of brotherly connection when I was young will never be fulfilled by a sexual relationship with a man, and that precludes me from leading a gay life."

  — Charles, 25, France and Turkey, page 65

- "It was incredibly liberating to come to understand that my attraction to other men at its core wasn't because of homosexuality *per se* but because of a deeper unmet need for me to connect with masculinity in order to complete my own growth."

  — Mohamed, 34, United Kingdom, Muslim, page 54

11

# Not Our True Selves

A number of men experienced a general sense that "gay" was not a core, authentic identity for them. It just didn't "fit" with their true sense of self, or it simply didn't feel right, morally. For example:

- "It was in conflict with my authentic self. It didn't make sense to me that God would create me to be gay."

    — "Rob," 47, California, page 97

- "Though same-sex attraction was never a choice, I have always felt that it was in conflict with the person that I truly am."

    — Charles, 40, Ohio, page 69

- "Homosexuality was already not working for me, but now [after my spiritual conversion] it also conflicted with my conviction that homosexual acts are immoral."

    — Tim, 37, Idaho, page 45

- "I never felt 100% at home during the time I lived that lifestyle. It never seemed to fit with who I am made to be, but I had addictive drives to continue the behaviors, even though they made me feel guilty and shameful. Since beginning the journey out of sexualized same-sex attraction, I have found more peace and satisfaction than I ever thought possible."

    — Robert, 47, Texas, page 76

- "My same-sex attractions did not resonate with the way I wanted to live my life. Part of the motivation was spiritual. Part of it was societal. But mainly, homosexuality just wasn't working for me."

    — "Monty," 24, New York, page 86

# General Dissatisfaction and a Desire to be Happier, Better

A lot of men described a general sense of overall unhappiness with life and a general desire to find greater peace and fulfillment. Some also described a yearning to simply be a better man, to become their best self—and for them, that didn't fit with their same-sex attractions.

- "My life was rapidly deteriorating. My mental health was suffering. I was depressed, anxious and had panic attacks. I had lost contact with my family. I was riddled with inner conflicts and was extremely unhappy as a result. I knew that I was living an unhealthy lifestyle that I had to change."

    — "Hakim," 24, United Arab Emirates, page 77

- "I want to change because I want to find the joy that I have not glimpsed in the gay environment. I firmly believe that what I want and really need is to fulfill my needs in healthy non-sexual ways."

    — Jose, 26, Mexico, page 78

- "I believed that by working to reduce the intensity of my homosexual attractions, I would be able to live my life with less stress and depression."

    — Kevin, 29, Idaho, page 49

- "When I was living a gay life, I felt this emptiness in my heart. I didn't know where it was coming from, but I realized that I needed to change. I realized that what I wanted most in my life was not to feel alone—but contrary to what everyone was telling me, pursuing a gay life style made me feel even more alone."

    — Stephan, 34, Germany, page 58

- "My real motivation is that I deserve to be happy, less burdened, more loved and cared for. I deserve to not be chained to what was done to me when I was younger. I also am motivated as a future father. I want to start a new path to a different kind of environment for my future children."

— Jeddy, 29, Texas, page 53

- "I felt that I wasn't reaching my potential. I felt that my body was naturally created heterosexual (physically, biologically, endocrinologically) but my psychology wasn't in step. I wanted more from life. Marriage. Children. To reach my fullest potential as a human male."

— Mohamed, 34, United Kingdom, page 54

- "I didn't like the man I became when I was with gay boyfriends or at their parties. In contrast, when I met [my future wife], I felt uplifted, like I was being called to be a better man. I liked the man I saw reflected in her eyes. That's who I really wanted to be."

— Rich, 53, Virginia, page 106

# Shame Never Motivates Real Change

What you don't see in these responses are significant references to outside pressure to change or fear of family or societal rejection for being gay—the kinds of things that most critics assume could only be motivating someone to pursue change.

In fact, when People Can Change surveyed member of our online support groups in 2006 about what factors were motivating their desire to reduce or eliminate their same-sex attractions, only 22% cited "outside pressure from others" as a major motivating factor. And while 74% did report experiencing *some* level of pressure or encouragement to *reject* their homosexuality, this was largely counter-balanced by 54% who also reported feeling some level of pressure or encouragement to *accept* their homosexuality.

Any successful change effort—whether we are talking about sexual attractions or weight loss or quitting smoke or earning a PhD—must be intrinsically self-motivated. In the long-term, people don't make difficult, lasting changes to please others. Change must always be authentically self-motivated.

And even more important, change efforts must not be based on shame. Shame may raise awareness of a need to change or the benefits of pursuing change. But shame alone can never motivate real change.

Quite the contrary. Successful change efforts of any kind must be built on a foundation of self-worth. We pursue change (of any kind) not to *become* good or worthy, but because we already *are* good and worthy—and therefore we deserve better for our future than we've had in the past. That's why People Can Change's Journey Into Manhood program teaches:

"If you gain nothing else from this weekend, we want you to know two truths:

"1. You are valuable and good just as you are — today, unchanged, and even if you never change.
"2. You have brothers who see your 'shadows' and accept you, just as you are."[3]

And:

"It seems ironic — but many men who have walked this journey out of homosexuality ahead of you have found that, until we could begin to love and accept ourselves just as we were, right then, unchanged, we could make little progress. Acceptance of our goodness, our value and our true potential was a critical early step out of homosexuality."[4]

---

[3] From the Journey Into Manhood program by People Can Change
[4]   http://www.peoplecanchange.com/change/notshame.php

13

# Our Lives Now

The difference in the before-and-after "pictures" of our lives—these then-and-now descriptions—could hardly be starker.

When People Can Change asked, ***"How would you rate the degree of your same-sex versus opposite-sex attractions currently?"*** almost half of respondents (47%) said they now experience themselves as either "exclusively heterosexual" or "primarily heterosexual, but with incidental homosexual attractions." Only 1% had said they fit one of those categories before.

Another way to look at these responses is that 90% said they were more homosexual than heterosexual "then"—at the time when their SSA was the most intense—with 43% describing themselves as exclusively homosexual at the time. Now, only 39% said they are more homosexual than heterosexual, with only 6% describing themselves as still exclusively homosexual.

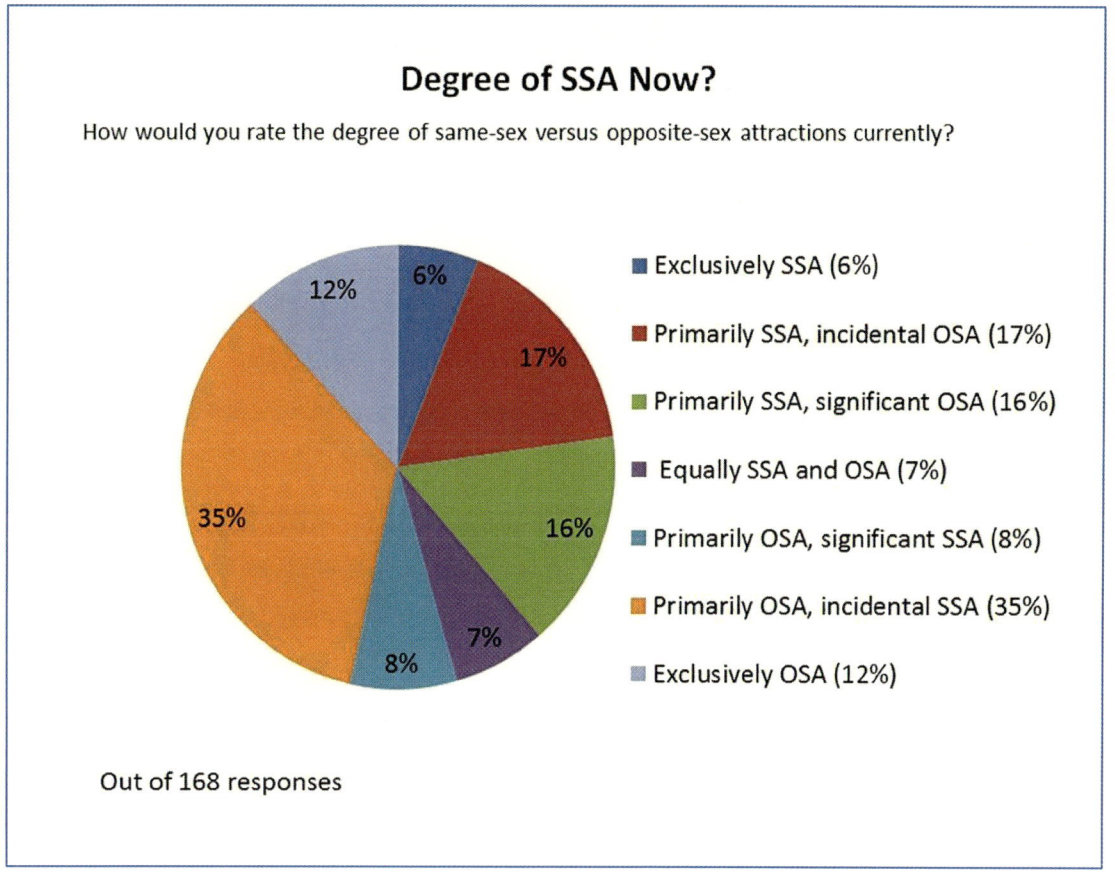

**Degree of SSA Now?**

How would you rate the degree of same-sex versus opposite-sex attractions currently?

- Exclusively SSA (6%)
- Primarily SSA, incidental OSA (17%)
- Primarily SSA, significant OSA (16%)
- Equally SSA and OSA (7%)
- Primarily OSA, significant SSA (8%)
- Primarily OSA, incidental SSA (35%)
- Exclusively OSA (12%)

Out of 168 responses

Clearly, these men perceive significant shifts (collectively) in their same-sex attractions.

*The pie charts in this book present a profile of those who responded to the People Can Change questionnaire from which the 54 brief summaries were drawn. They do not indicate representative samplings of SSA or gay populations or of all those who have attempted sexual-orientation changes.*

The next question asked about "same-sex sexual or romantic *behaviors* or relationships." This is about what the men *did*, not about what they *felt*.

Out of 171 respondents, 78% said they experienced either a complete, major or moderate reduction in SSA behaviors and relationships. This is in addition to another 9% who reported never having acted on their SSA physically or interpersonally either before or since (and thus, no reduction could be reported).

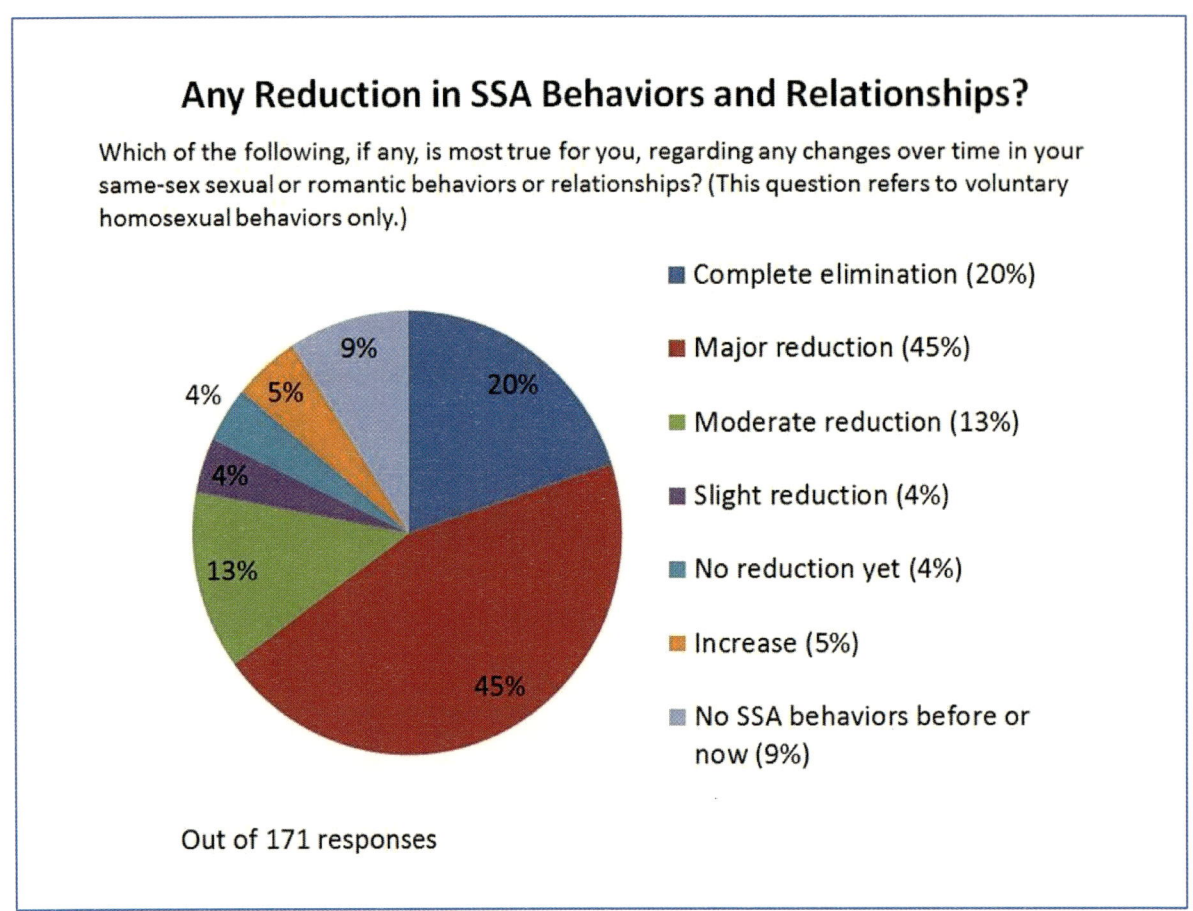

**Any Reduction in SSA Behaviors and Relationships?**

Which of the following, if any, is most true for you, regarding any changes over time in your same-sex sexual or romantic behaviors or relationships? (This question refers to voluntary homosexual behaviors only.)

- Complete elimination (20%)
- Major reduction (45%)
- Moderate reduction (13%)
- Slight reduction (4%)
- No reduction yet (4%)
- Increase (5%)
- No SSA behaviors before or now (9%)

Out of 171 responses

This seems especially significant given the number of men who related in their personal narratives how addictively or compulsively they had sought out homosexual encounters, relationships, or pornography in their earlier lives.

16

Sometimes even the most ardent opponents of sexual-orientation change efforts will concede that, sure, some people can change their behavior and get sexually sober or become celibate, but that doesn't mean the attraction itself has diminished, they say.

So the next question asked specifically about changes in the attractions themselves. This question was about what the men *feel*, not about what they *do*.

Out of 173 respondents, 83% said they experienced either a complete, major or moderate reduction in SSA feelings, attractions and desires.

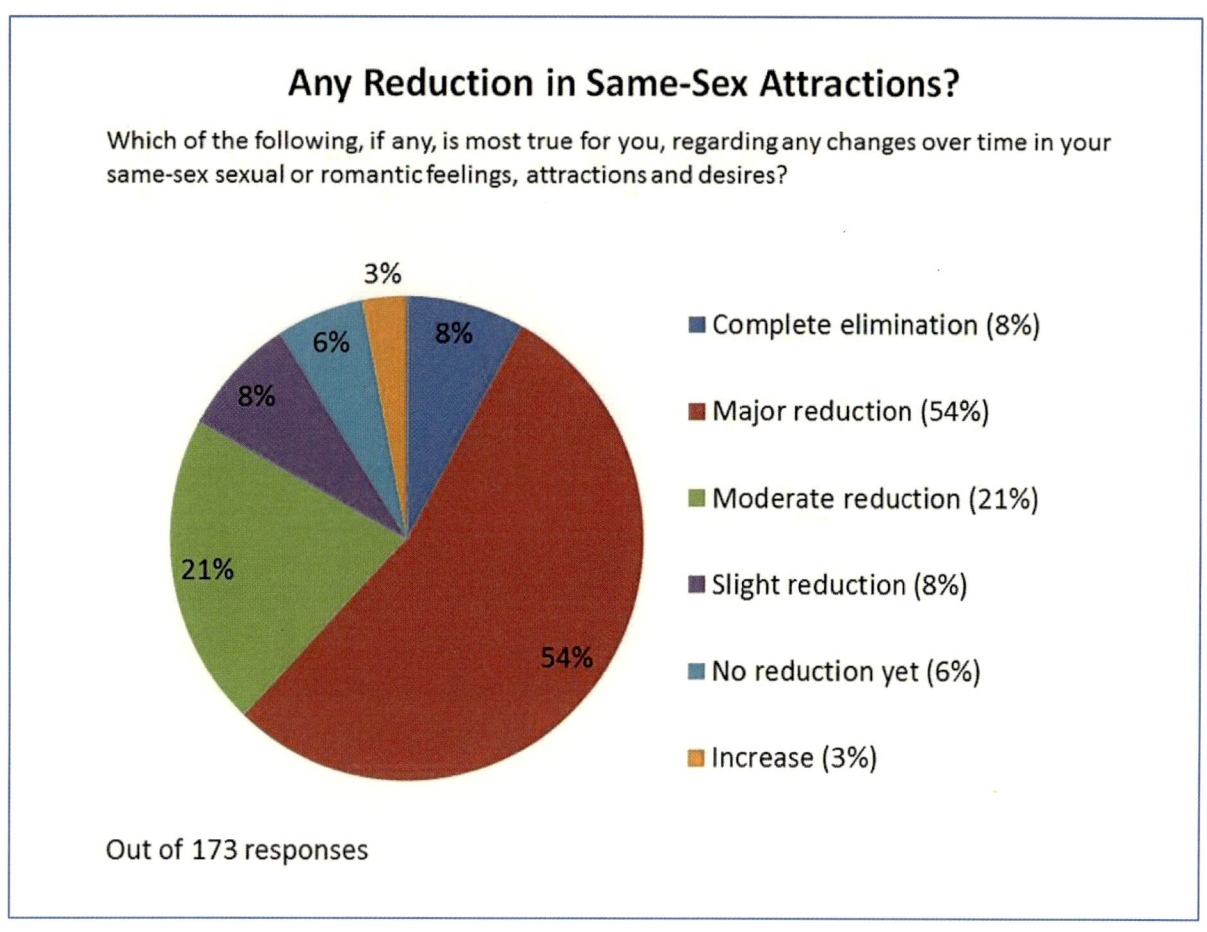

What about opposite-sex attractions and heterosexual behaviors like dating and marriage?

It's important to realize that not everyone who seeks to reduce their same-sex attractions is necessarily concerned about developing opposite-sex attractions. Some men do, of course—they sincerely want to marry a woman, have children and a happy marriage and home life together. But other men simply want the inner turmoil of SSA to go away; whether heterosexual feelings emerge or increase is less important—or even irrelevant to them.

Nevertheless, according to the men we questioned, more than half (59%) experienced a complete, major or moderate increase in opposite-sex attractions.

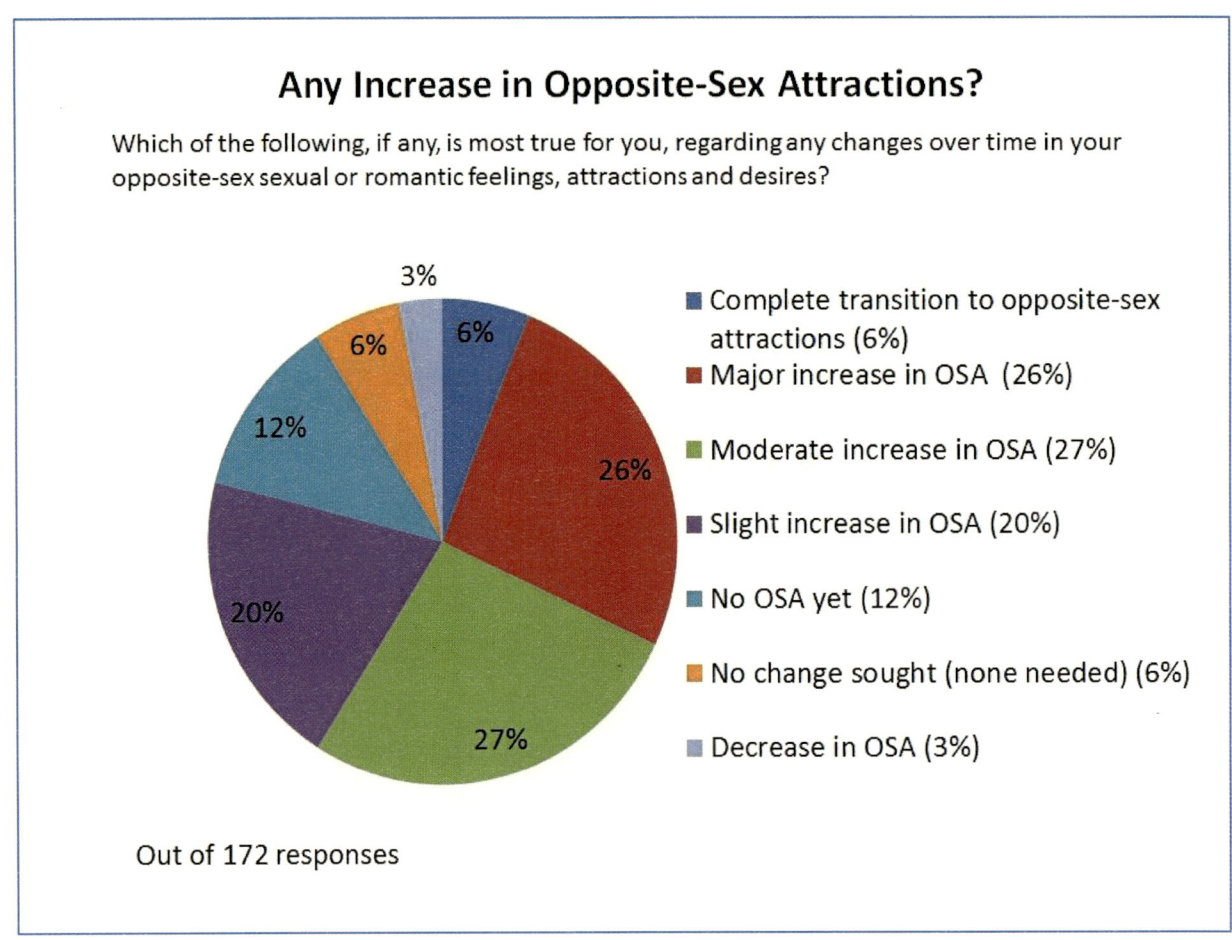

**Any Increase in Opposite-Sex Attractions?**

Which of the following, if any, is most true for you, regarding any changes over time in your opposite-sex sexual or romantic feelings, attractions and desires?

3%
6%
6%
12%
26%
20%
27%

- Complete transition to opposite-sex attractions (6%)
- Major increase in OSA (26%)
- Moderate increase in OSA (27%)
- Slight increase in OSA (20%)
- No OSA yet (12%)
- No change sought (none needed) (6%)
- Decrease in OSA (3%)

Out of 172 responses

For almost as many respondents (56%), those increased attractions also translated to increased heterosexual behaviors and relationships.

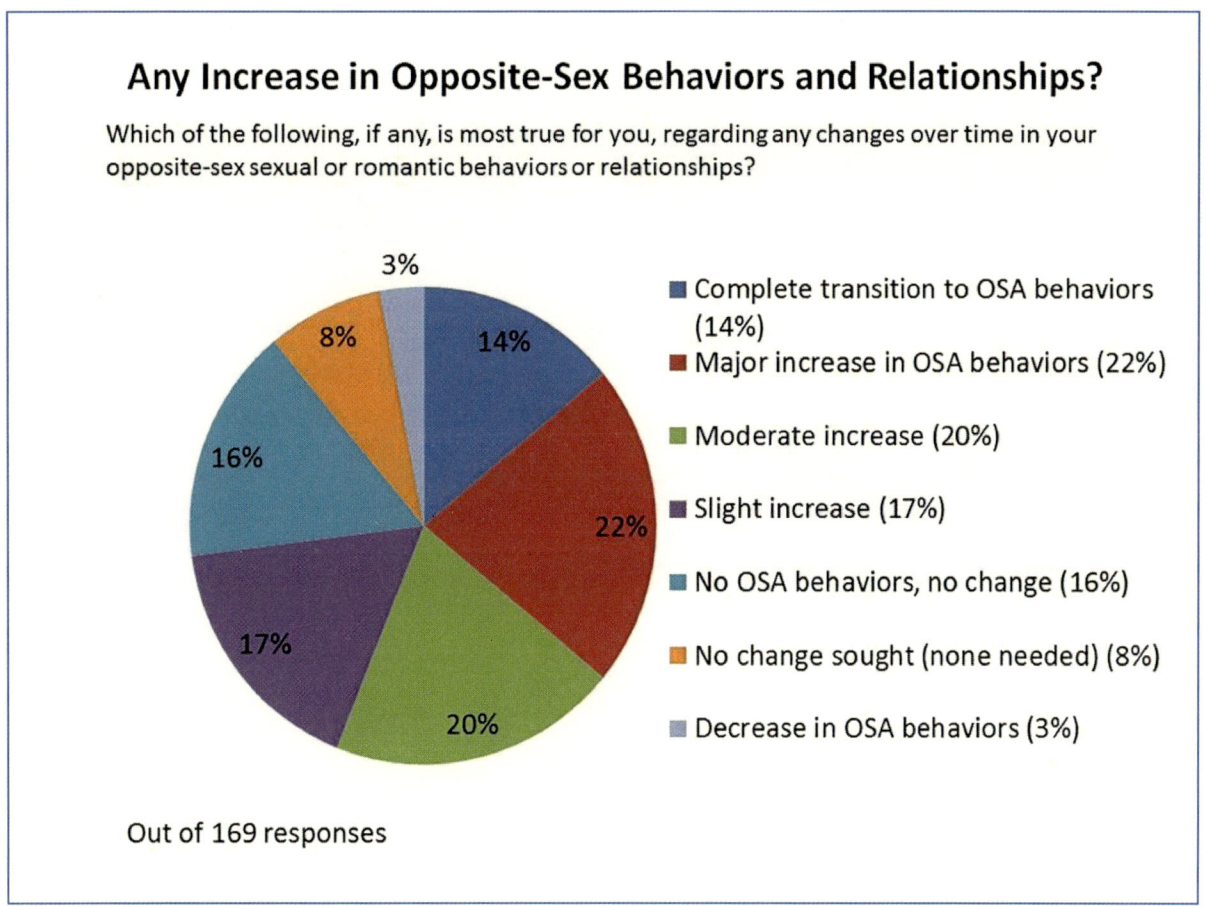

## How Much Change?

So how much sexual-orientation change is reasonable to expect?

That, of course, can never be predicted for any particular individual. In any type of therapy or self-improvement program, there can never be any guaranteed outcomes—and sexual-orientation change efforts are no different. If anything, change is more difficult, because we are dealing with something as primal and powerful as our sexuality. But it is informative to look at the profiles of the men who responded to the People Can Change questionnaire to see how much change they report experiencing.

Remember that People Can Change asked respondents to rate their sexual attractions on a range of seven possible options:

- Exclusively *homo*sexual
- Primarily *homo*sexual but with incidental *hetero*sexual attractions
- Primarily *homo*sexual but with significant *hetero*sexual attractions
- About equally heterosexual and homosexual
- Primarily *hetero*sexual but with significant *homo*sexual attractions
- Primarily *hetero*sexual but with incidental *homo*sexual attractions
- Exclusively *hetero*sexual.

This is essentially what's known as a Kinsey Scale, or a Heterosexual-Homosexual Rating Scale, which was developed by psychologist Alfred Kinsey in the 1940s.

In the questionnaire, People Can Change asked men to rate their attractions at two different points in their lives: At the time when their SSA was the most intense, and currently. We then compared how much shift the respondents collectively reported.

- The most frequent response, reported by more than a fifth (22%) of respondents, indicated that their attractions had moved **one** level on the seven-point scale—say, from "exclusively homosexual" to "primarily homosexual but with *incidental* heterosexual attractions," or from that point to "primarily homosexual but with *significant* heterosexual attractions." Like this:

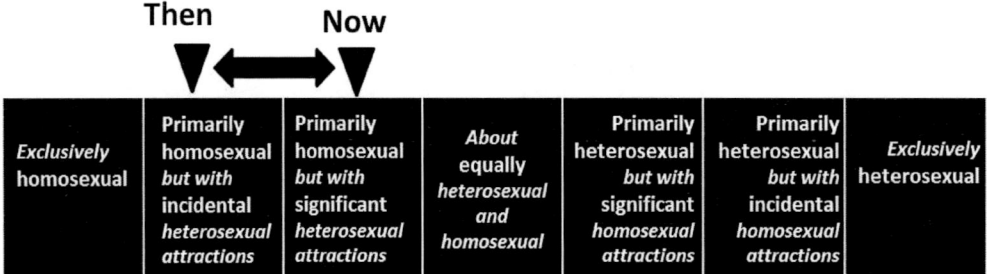

- The next most frequently response, reported by almost as many (19%), indicated **four** levels of change on the Kinsey scale, such as:

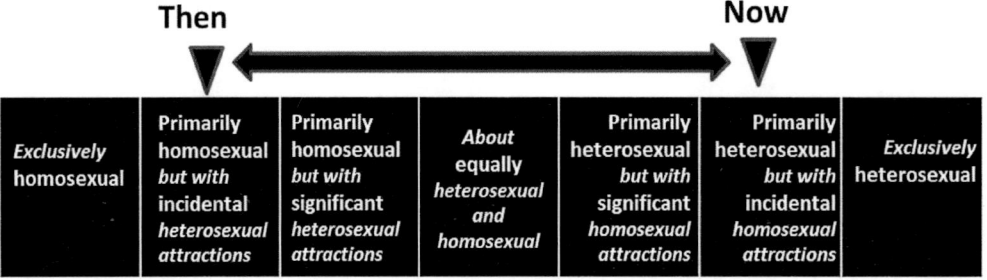

- The *least* common response—from five out of 163 men, or 3% of respondents—was from those who indicated their attractions had shifted all **six** levels, from "exclusively homosexual" to "exclusively heterosexual." This was the most extreme and least common degree of reported change in sexual attractions—and, frankly, least likely to occur.

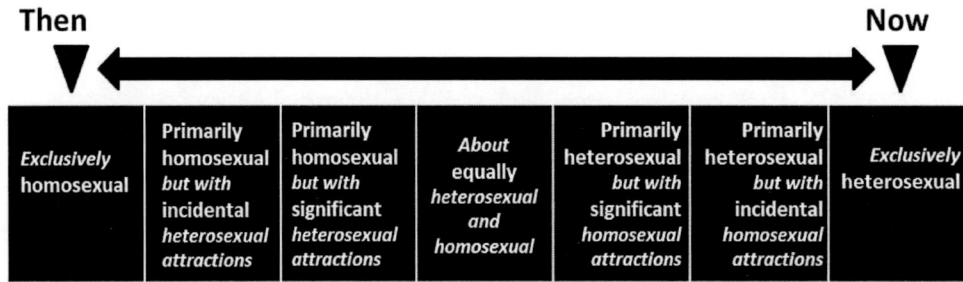

- About 16% reported no change—they rated their attractions as being at the same point on the seven-point scale both "then" and "now."

  — About a third of this subgroup said they were exclusively homosexual both then and now.

  — More than a third said they were "primarily homosexual but with incidental heterosexual attractions" at both points in time.

  — The rest rated themselves further to the right on the scale, but still the same at both points in time.

Here's another way to look at these responses:

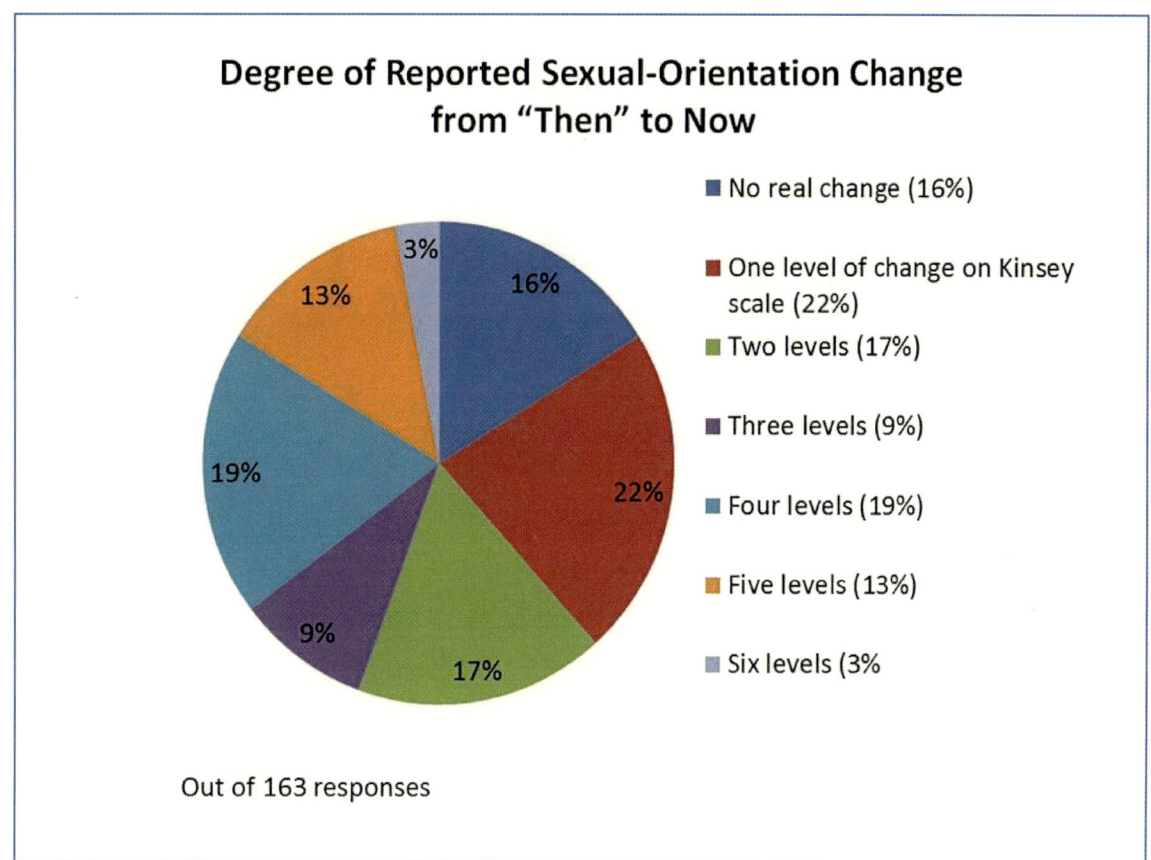

**Degree of Reported Sexual-Orientation Change from "Then" to Now**

- No real change (16%)
- One level of change on Kinsey scale (22%)
- Two levels (17%)
- Three levels (9%)
- Four levels (19%)
- Five levels (13%)
- Six levels (3%

Out of 163 responses

Again, this is not a prediction of what any particular individual will experience. But the experience of these 163 respondents can help set realistic expectations of how much, if any, change in sexual orientation is likely to occur.

And here's another disclaimer: Most men dealing with same-sex attractions dislike labeling themselves or attempting to quantify the degree and intensity of their sexual feelings. By its very nature, sexuality is too nuanced to fit into a box or even on a seven-point scale. Here, we have nonetheless reduced complex life experiences and feelings to scales and tables and labels only to provide context, help set expectations, and even just to make it possible to communicate about this sensitive subject.

Besides, people inevitably pursue sexual-orientation change as a means to an end, not an end in itself. The real end goal typically is to find peace, wholeness, brotherly love, alignment with God's will, or improved family life. And on that front, there is little question of the success, for so many people, of their change efforts.

## Happier, More at Peace, Greater Self-Esteem

The men who responded to the People Can Change questionnaire and who share their stories in this book describe a degree of peace, happiness and improved self-esteem they had not experienced before:

- "I am now living the way that I want and am the happiest I have been in a very long time. …After lots of work, my SSA no longer has the intense grip that it once had on me."

  — Jason, 22, Utah, page 43

- "Therapy and healing weekends have not only helped me to see my problems differently but to see myself as someone who is good and valuable and acceptable just as I am—even unchanged."

  — Jose, 26, Mexico, page 78

- "I have also experienced major healing for emotional wounds and have seen every aspect of my life improve over the last three years."

  — Jeremy, 36, Texas, page 39

- "My efforts never were to change my sexual orientation but to be happy as the man I am—the man God created me to be. I've seen an increase in my self-esteem and renewed confidence. I have much more joy in my life. … My love for [my wife] has increased a lot. I'm more secure and confident as a father, too."

  — Stephan, 34, Germany, page 58

- "Emotionally I am a much healthier person. I used to have really deep emotional lows, to the point that I considered suicide several times. Now, I am happy. I like myself, where before I did not. My self-esteem is much greater than it has ever been. I feel respected and appreciated by men, where before I felt merely tolerated (or downright rejected) by them. My marriage is very strong. I love her more deeply than ever. I feel masculine; before I did not. I feel like an adult; before I felt like an 8-year-old boy stuck in a 48-year-old body of a man."

  — Scott, 51, Iowa, page 52

## More Authentically Connected to the World of Men

They describe themselves as grounded in their own sense of the masculine, and more connected as brothers to the greater world of men at large.

- "I don't have same-sex attractions today in the sense that when I see a good-looking guy I don't want to engage with him in any sort of sexual way. I see him as an equal—a brother with good and bad qualities, just like me."

  — Mohamed, 34, United Kingdom, page 54

- "I have learned that I need intimate, healthy, emotionally connected relationships with other men. As I have taken the steps to be open and vulnerable with the men in my life, I am growing in these relationships. This is filling the void in my heart that I used to medicate with gay porn or acting out sexually with other men. The real connection I long for with other men is not sexual or romantic, but pure, brotherly affection, affirmation and belonging."

  — "Richard," 45, Oregon, page 73

- "I found the ex-gay community and it seemed to better represent my identity as a man with same-sex attraction. These people help me feel whole and masculine. They help me to understand and successfully maintain healthy boundaries to meet my needs."

  — Maurice, 36, Alabama, page 60

- "My sexual attractions to guys are far less than they used to be. They happen less often and are not as strong. I still find men attractive, but the desires are desires to be friends, to get to know each other, to somehow become more like what I see in him. There's not nearly as much of that same needy, clingy desperate feeling. I find that my brotherly male friendships bring an incredible sense of joy and peace into my life. Sexual connection or exclusive relationship scenarios fade in the light of the joy I feel with my brothers."

— Benjamin, 37, California, page 93

- "My same-sex attraction is modestly diminished, but far more importantly, I am comfortable with that as a part of who I am, open about it with my friends, and have mostly found a way to get those needs for intimacy met with men through non-sexual outlets."

— "Yaakov," 37, California, page 87

- "I never 'acted out' before, so that hasn't changed, but now I feel much more on equal grounds with other men."

— Tim, 48, Oregon, page 56

## Sexual Behaviors More Aligned With Values

They frequently describe their "acting out" (sexual behaviors that are "out of bounds" for their own personal moral code or values) as having diminished significantly—or sometimes completely.

- "I have not acted out with another man in over three years and do not have the desire to pursue men sexually or to view pornography."

— Jeremy, 36, Texas, page 39

- "I am no longer acting out on my pornography addiction, and this has greatly helped me and my desires. Today, my SSA feelings are significantly less than they were before. Now, when they come up, I can deal with them in healthy ways and in ways that make me feel good about myself afterward."

— Sam, 26, Utah, page 47

- "I no longer experience shame or guilt around my homosexual attractions. I do not experience any conflict between my attractions and my personal value system. I do not feel sexually repressed or incomplete because I am not actively expressing my homosexuality. I believe I am in a situation equal to any individual who is in a committed relationship with one individual and yet still experiences attractions to other individuals."

— Kevin, 29, Idaho, page 49

- "I have been able to let go if the insatiable need to 'act out' sexually. I have learned tools to dissolve SSA feelings and work within boundaries of healthy friendships."

— Stephen, 41, Texas, page 90

- "It has been over 14 years since I've had any sexual behavior with other men and at least 10 years since I've even wanted to. My desire for a homosexual romantic relationship is completely gone, and now I desire to have a romantic relationship with a woman."

— Tim, 37, Idaho, page 45

# More Attracted to Women

Some of the men who shared their stories for this book describe a degree of attraction to or affection for women that they never thought was possible.

- "I have had no interest in dating other men since 2003. Currently, I am very happy and functional in a heterosexual relationship. Romantic feelings toward my girlfriend were present immediately when we met, and the sexual desires I have toward her are equal to those I once had for men when I was pursuing a homosexual lifestyle. With her, I feel genuinely and completely fulfilled emotionally, spiritually, and sexually."

  — David, 41, Arizona, page 72

- "Today I feel very grounded in my male identity and definitely see women as something different from what I am. My sexual impulses for women are minimal, but relationally I love interacting and partnering with them as people who are at their essence different from who I am."

  — Tim, 48, Oregon, page 56

- "In bed with my wife, my focus is mainly on her—how much I desire her, how much I love her, how much I want to please her. Sexual relations with her have increased dramatically. At one point I really did not have sexual desire for her. Now I can't seem to keep my hands off of her."

  — Scott, 51, Iowa, page 52

- "My marriage is better than I could have dreamed, and my wife is now my best friend."

  — Chuck, 56, Florida, page 88

- "My SSA is gone. I have no desire to have sex with men. I am strongly attracted to having sex with women and look forward to it with great excitement."

  — Sean, 60, Arizona, page 96

- "My SSA has been greatly reduced. There are days when it seems non-existent. I have noticed that when my SSA is reduced, my opposite-sex attractions naturally increase."

  — "Jerry," 43, Maryland, page 102

# Numerous Benefits Not Directly Related to SSA

The People Can Change questionnaire asked, *"As a result of your sexual-orientation change efforts, have you experienced benefits not directly related to your sexual attractions?"*

The responses were numerous and varied, but many men mentioned:

1. Improved self-esteem overall.

2. More self-confidence.

3. An increased connection to their own internal sense of masculinity—an enhanced sense of pride and confidence in being a man.

4. More friendships, and more meaningful friendships, with greater (non-sexual) intimacy.

5. A new marriage, sometimes, or a much-improved marriage, and better family relationships overall.

6. Greater sense of living authentically, without hiding or pretending.

7. Feeling closer to God.

Here is how some men describe these changes (for more, see responses in the "Any Other Benefits?" row of each of the 54 brief summaries).

- "Certainly, here is where I felt change through the roof. My confidence in who I am as a man, my ability to stand up and speak my truth and be heard, my letting go of defining myself by SSA or anything else, my leadership abilities, care of others, and soundness of mind have grown enormously. I would not be the secure leader and man that I am today if it wasn't for this work."

  — Tim, 48, Oregon, page 56

- "Yes, I have seen every aspect of my life improve. I feel a lot more assertive and confident at work and in all of my personal relationships. This has made me a much more effective leader and enabled me to be much more effective in my relationships with family and friends. Everyone has noticed a major improvement. I am happier than I've ever been."

  — Jeremy, 36, Texas, page 39

- "I have had huge benefits unrelated to my unwanted SSA. I have become a man with self-esteem, integrity, and confidence. I am able to be a better husband, father, son, employer and human being. I understand my masculinity and am able to express it. I have honest, open and meaningful friendships that are based on who and what I truly am. I am happy and I help bring joy to those around me. This is not at all who I was before this work."

  — Steve, 55, Florida, page 103

- "I have learned to assert myself and to not allow myself to be taken advantage of. I have improved as a husband and father, with incredible confidence. I have learned to relate to other men as a man among men, rather than seeing myself as less-than or unworthy of masculine love and affirmation. I feel like a man, and for the first time in my life, I am actually thankful to be a man."

  — Charles, 40, Ohio, page 69

## SSA Can Still Return Under Stress

Despite all the progress, many men say their same-sex attractions still "show up" when they are distressed or don't get their basic emotional needs met, especially needs for healthy, non-sexual male bonding.

- "When I experience increased SSA, it alerts me to a problem area in my life that I need to address. When I deal with that lack, the SSA again subsides. The strength of my SSA indicates to me how much of a man I feel I am, at a given moment. When I make the choices that are conducive to my psychological well-being, then I can go without experiencing any SSA whatsoever. Instead I experience identification with other men, and consequently experience increased opposite-sex attraction. When I'm not doing what I need to do for self-care, again I notice the appearance of SSA."

  — Hakim, 24, United Arab Emirates, page 77

- "Occasionally, when I feel insecure or emotionally hurt, I may find myself having sexual feelings toward men. I have learned to go back to the root cause and address it. …My SSA today happens occasionally when I am triggered emotionally by events at work that make me feel insecure about myself as a man."

  — Robert, 47, Texas, page 76

- The only times when same-sex sexual feelings attractions and desires start to creep back into my life are when I feel I am unable to connect with men in a healthy, non-sexual way.

  — Scott, 51, Iowa, page 52

# If Sexual Attractions Don't Change

But what happens to those who try to alter or reduce their sexual attractions and are not successful at it?

Among those who responded to the People Can Change questionnaire, 16% (25 men out of 163) reported no significant change in their sexual attractions between "then" and now. Some critics contend that this kind of outcome can cause so much depression, anxiety or self-recrimination that it's better never to make the attempt to begin with.

This makes no sense to us. Let's say we're talking about an unwanted sexual *behavior* rather than an unwanted sexual *feeling*—a behavior like pornography use, for example. Would anyone seriously argue that it's best for a man to *not even try* to reduce or eliminate from his life the pornography that is causing him such distress? After all, he might not succeed at the effort, and then he might suffer from even more depression and self-criticism!

No, it's often better to make the effort (assuming one is intrinsically self-motived to try), but to build on a solid foundation of self-esteem, regardless of the outcome. (See "Shame Never Motivates Real Change," page 13.) We pursue self-improvement (of any kind) not to *become* good or worthy, but because we already *are* good and worthy— and as such, we deserve better for our future than we've had in the past.

Even among the 25 men who answered the People Can Change questionnaire by saying that their same-sex attractions were basically the same now as they were before, only two or three reported significantly negative feelings and experiences (see Section 5, "Any Harm?," page 31). The rest reported very positive life changes and personal growth as a result of the work they have done, despite the lack of change in their sexual attractions.[5]

- "I've been doing this for 20 years. I've never even kissed a guy and still don't feel like I'm missing out. A gay life would have caused more pain and hurt for me and would conflict with my deep-rooted boundaries. All my change efforts and resources have helped me to be a better person. I've especially benefited from the recognition that underneath all these problems and addictions are legitimate needs."

  — "Jay," 42, Utah

- "I have had no negative effects from change efforts. Just the opposite. I considered both change and gay-affirmative options to be a difficult challenge, with potential risks. Doing nothing wasn't an option for me any longer, but gay-affirmation seemed much more radical and permanent. I considered the change option to be more measured and reversible if it didn't work for me."

  — "Yaakov," 37, California, page 87

- "I've felt frustration with my progress. But I was in far more depression and loneliness prior to seeking help and change."

  — "JR," 23, California

- "I have come to accept the fact that I have SSA and that doesn't make me a horrible person. I have experienced acceptance from others who know about my SSA. I am actually thankful for this trial and see the good that can come out of it."

  — "Francisco," 20, Kansas

- "Even though my sexual attractions haven't really diminished, I have more self-esteem and self-assurance. I feel better about myself in general and I've been able to step into many tasks powerfully, where I was afraid to do that before. I'm a leader and a mentor in my community."

  — Justin, 33, Israel

As you read the 50-plus first-person accounts that follow, you'll see that, even among those who have experienced relatively minimal change in their sexual attractions, they've still experienced dramatic growth in other important areas of their lives.

---

[5] Just remember, these are not random survey results and cannot be projected onto everyone who has ever attempted change. The point is, change efforts like these can still be extremely helpful—even life-saving—for many, even if they don't achieve the degree or type of change originally hoped for.

# What Brought About These Changes?

If all you heard about <u>reparative therapy</u> or other sexual-orientation change efforts was what you Googled and read on gay-activist blogs and mainstream media, you could easily conclude—erroneously—that change therapies and change programs invariably are forced on young people against their will.[6] You might also believe—mistakenly—that these programs are shame-based, are hostile and homophobic, and use aversion therapies up to and including electric shock treatments. Or, at the other extreme, you might conclude—again, erroneously—that they represent religious extremism that relies on nothing but prayer. ("Pray away the gay" is a clever mockery-turned-campaign slogan coined by opponents, but no known advocate believes it or would ever use that phrase.)

All these claims are rampant on the Internet. Not because they are facts, but because they are talking points. Not because they are science, but because they further an ideological agenda. (Remember: "…if you repeat [a lie] frequently enough, people will sooner or later believe it."[7])

In stark contrast to these claims are real-world experiences like those shared by the 54 men in this book. How could force, shaming, hostility or aversion therapies possibly yield the kinds of life changes described in this book? How could they possibly result in improved self-esteem, greater self-confidence, an enhanced sense of masculinity, better friendships, more authentic self-expression, greater peace, happier marriages, and so on?

The answer is they couldn't. Because those alleged tactics—those lies—are nothing like what authentic sexual-orientation change efforts are really about.

The <u>People Can Change</u> questionnaire asked, ***"What brought about any changes you described above in your same-sex attractions over time?"*** and ***"What kinds of support, help or intervention, if any, did you pursue (or have you pursued)?"***

Respondents emphasized about 10 areas of significant healing and personal growth work that benefited them.

1.  Engaging in deep emotional-healing work through therapy or counseling, or through intensive experiential-healing workshops, or both. Uncovering and healing underlying emotional issues and resolving emotional pain from the past.

2.  Discovering and meeting underlying emotional needs, especially for non-sexual, brotherly (or fatherly) affection, affirmation and bonding.

3.  Increasing self-acceptance, self-confidence, assertiveness and self-esteem.

4.  Overcoming shame.

5.  Anchoring a deeper sense of masculinity and confidence in being a man.

6.  Building healthy, non-sexual, secure male friendships and a sense of belonging to safe communities of men.

7.  Becoming sexually sober (meaning abstinent from dissonant or out-of-control sexual behaviors).

8.  Growing in spirituality.

---

[6] For example, people often assume that participants in People Can Change's Journey Into Manhood program are primarily in their teens or early 20s. In fact, the average age of participants is 36, and the minimum is 18. Journey Into Manhood does not accept minors.
[7] Psychoanalyst Walter Langer

9. Becoming more authentic, honest and "real" in relationships with others.

10. Building meaningful support networks, and receiving authentic support from friends, wives, mentors, religious leaders and others.

Some of the most frequently mentioned resources or tools were:

1. The Journey Into Manhood experiential weekend program by People Can Change.[8]

2. Therapists or counselors who are supportive of the individual's desire to explore sexual-orientation change, and especially those who are experienced and skilled in sexual-orientation change therapies.

3. Supportive religious ministries, like the former Exodus[9] organization in the U.S. (Christian/Protestant), Courage (Catholic), Evergreen or North Star (LDS or Mormon), and JONAH (Jewish).

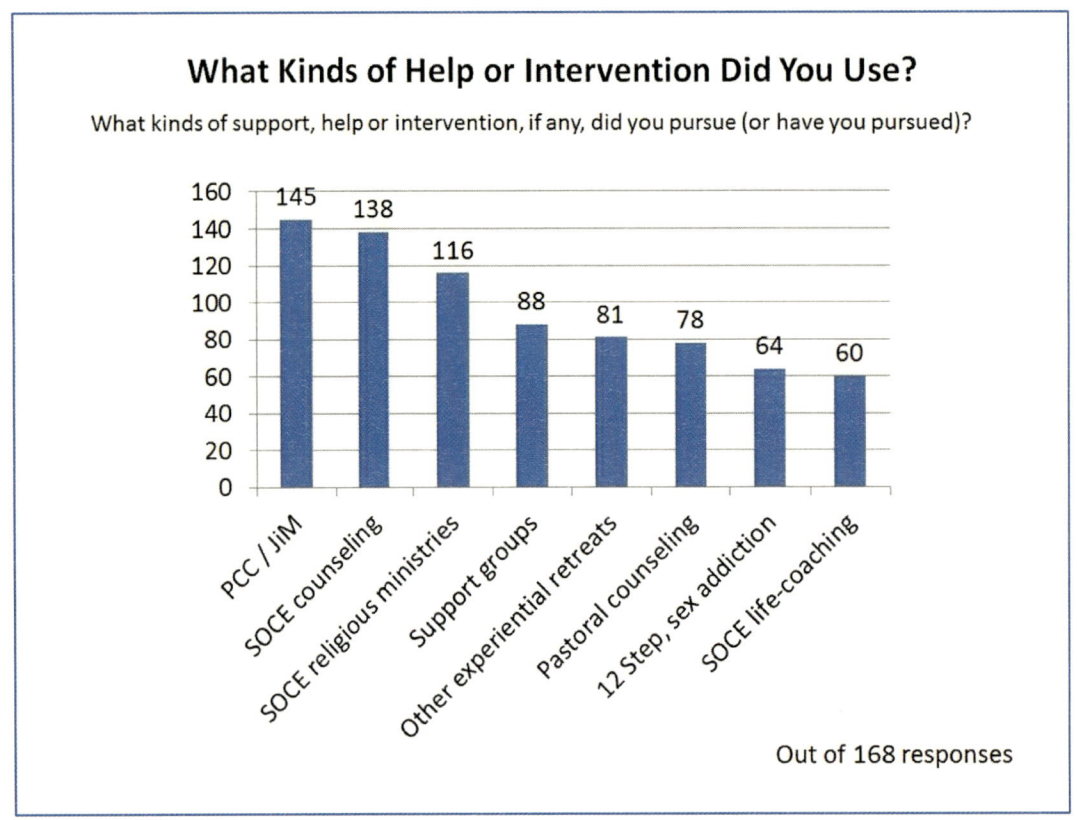

4. Support groups, including religiously based support groups and local follow-up groups from Journey Into Manhood (called MANS groups) or follow-up online/phone support.

5. Other experiential-healing or personal growth weekends by a variety of organizations, like New Warriors, Noble Man, Adventure In Manhood, Samson Society, Edge Venture, etc.

6. Pastoral counseling.

7. 12 Step programs like Sexaholics Anonymous, Sex Addicts Anonymous or Celebrate Recovery.

---

[8] These results are naturally skewed because so many of the men who were sent the questionnaire have participated in PCC's Journey Into Manhood program. A questionnaire sent to a broader audience would have ranked these programs differently.
[9] Succeeded by Restored Hope Network (http://restoredhopenetwork.org/)

8. Life-coaching with professionals who have experienced sexual-orientation change themselves.

9. Books on SSA-related recovery, or Bibliotherapy.

Following is a sampling of responses to the question, ***"What brought about any changes you described above in your same-sex attractions over time?"*** and the follow-up question, ***"What was most helpful or beneficial to you?"***

- "I've come to realize that this attraction is an emotional one for me. When my core emotional needs are met by men in healthy, non-sexual ways, my SSA automatically decreases."

  — "Jerry," 43, Maryland, page 102

- "Most helpful were reparative therapy; the New Warrior Training Adventure and follow-up groups; trusted, caring mentors; deep connections with new, trusted friends; getting sexually sober through Sexaholics Anonymous; and the support of a loving wife. All of this was guided by a deep spiritual connection and a humble submission to God's will for my life."

  — Rich, 53, Virginia, page 106

- "It was incredibly liberating to come to understand that my attraction to other men at its core wasn't because of homosexuality *per se* but because of a deeper unmet need for me to connect with masculinity in order to complete my own growth. I realized that interacting with men in a sexual way wasn't helping me attain masculinity within myself. It was futile. Like drinking salt water to quench a thirst."

  — Mohamed, 34, United Kingdom, page 54

- "[Most helpful was] individual counseling with a licensed mental health professional who was open to my choices. He was non-judgmental and would have supported me in whatever choice I made. The next most important thing was connection and positive association with other men in situations similar to mine."

  — Kevin, 29, Idaho, page 49

- "Most helpful for me was the love, acceptance and open conversations with my wife. But also the experiential weekend retreats from People Can Change made a significant difference. Because of them I was able to truly understand who I am and let go of all the shame and baggage in my life. I was able to understand what happened and how to push through all of it. Attending a local MANS Group gave me the platform to grow more. Finally, meeting with a counselor and therapist gave me the tools to push through everything from my past that was still there."

  — Stephan, 34, Germany, page 58

- "I realized that my homosexual desires were pointing to what I really wanted and needed—authentic connection with other men. I began to nourish authentic male friendships in my everyday life. … [Most helpful was] realizing that first I had to accept myself just the way I was, then realizing that nothing was wrong with me because of my homosexual attractions. I wasn't 'born that way'; the same-sex attractions came about because I didn't feel like I belonged in the world of men, and because I saw women as smothering, selfish, and needy. Then I was able to work on changing those beliefs instead of focusing on the homosexual attractions."

  — Tim, 37, Idaho, page 45

- "I attended Journey Into Manhood, which completely improved my self-esteem and concept of sexuality, due to the psychodramatic processes I experienced, but also because of the safe community of non-sexual male friendships I developed. I lost all shame for any prior behaviors and began to openly discuss my transformation with others. … I attended The Noble Man, an experiential weekend run by women, who helped me stop transferring my relationship with my mother onto my wife and most women I knew. I attended the New Warrior Training Adventure, which taught me how to communicate openly with men of all faiths and sexualities. I developed confidence to be the man I was intended to be. I now meet with my ManKind Project (New Warrior) brothers weekly, to continue healthy relationships with salient, encouraging men. They are straight, bi, and gay, and I love and trust each one with some of the most private and intimate details of my life."

— Chuck, 56, Florida, page 88

- "[Most helpful were] counseling, psychotherapy, and experiential trainings like <u>Journey Into Manhood</u> or other trainings concentrating on the development of my male identity. I learned to understand my emotions, deal with my emotions, show and share emotions. I learned to be authentic in relationships with men and women. I worked through traumatic experiences and distress. I learned to accept my own body and my own manhood. I learned to accept others, love others and to overcome fear."

— Stefan, 41, Germany, page 71

As anyone can see, those of us who share our stories in these 54 brief summaries (along with the 173 men who answered the questionnaire) experienced no such thing as electric shock therapies or other aversion tactics (which, in reality, have not been practiced in the Western world for 50 years or more). We experienced no shaming, no threats, no casting out of demons, no naïve and vastly oversimplified prescriptions for just "praying away the gay" (a slogan made up by opponents to change efforts, by the way).

No, what brought about real change for men like us started with building self-acceptance and self-worth, emotional-healing work, meeting core needs for emotional bonding with other men—and more. Some of it was hard work, but all of it ultimately was healing, affirming and constructive.

## Section Five:

# Any Harm?

After asking the men who responded to the <u>People Can Change</u> questionnaire about their lives now, and about any benefits they may have experienced from their sexual-orientation change efforts, the questionnaire followed up with, ***"What was less helpful, or even harmful?"*** The question was open-ended, not multiple choice. Those who responded volunteered their own answers.

Among everyone who answered the question, 35% said they experienced nothing harmful, while a combined 24% said they felt harmed by:

- Counselors who tried to push them to accept being gay.

- Unsupportive friends or family who rejected their change efforts and tried to persuade them to accept being gay.

- Overall cultural or community pressure to accept being gay.

That's a combined 59% whose only negative experience was feeling rejected or disrespected for not wanting to accepting a gay identity, and with it, pressure to live a gay life. Another 2% said their frustration was with the difficulty in finding a therapist who had any experience or skill in working with people who did not want to embrace homosexuality as an identity and lifestyle.

Other experiences that a small number of respondents reported as being less effective or even harmful included:

- Pastoral counseling, with often well-meaning but inexperienced religious counselors.

- Counseling overall, or a bad relationship with a particular counselor.

- Interpersonal conflicts or unhealthy or hurtful interpersonal relationships with friends, support group peers, and others.

- Bad experiences in particular ministries.

We've grouped responses from 25 men who volunteered a wide array of relatively isolated experiences into an "other" category in the following pie chart. These "other" responses describe experiences that were less effective, or even harmful, or that simply didn't work well for them, such as:

- "Acting out" sexually (four responses).

- Remaining in isolation, doing nothing about the SSA (three responses).

- Twelve step programs (two responses).

- Support groups (two responses).

- Over-intellectualizing, or too much introspection (one response).

- Over-spiritualizing what was, at its root, not really a spiritual problem (one response).

- Cost of therapy and other change programs (one response).

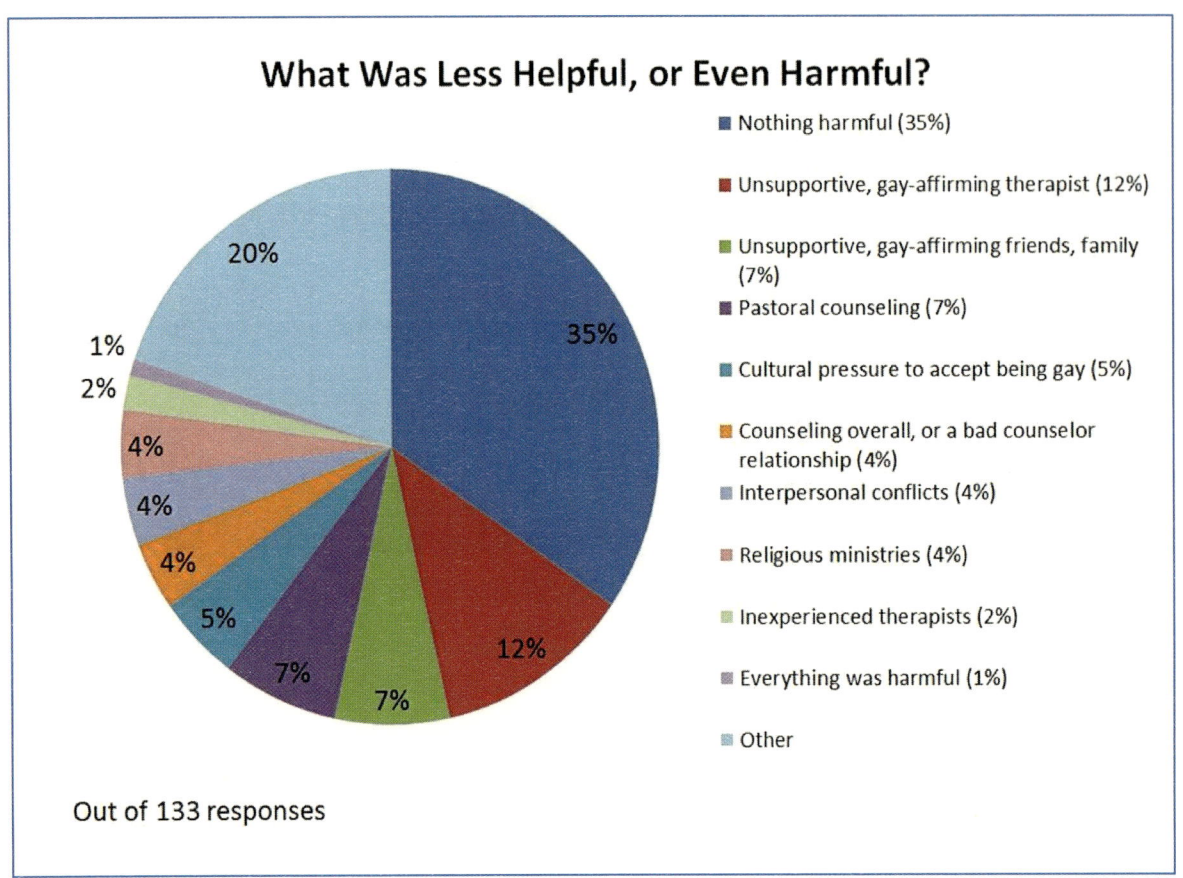

## What Was Less Helpful, or Even Harmful?

- ■ Nothing harmful (35%)
- ■ Unsupportive, gay-affirming therapist (12%)
- ■ Unsupportive, gay-affirming friends, family (7%)
- ■ Pastoral counseling (7%)
- ■ Cultural pressure to accept being gay (5%)
- ■ Counseling overall, or a bad counselor relationship (4%)
- ■ Interpersonal conflicts (4%)
- ■ Religious ministries (4%)
- ■ Inexperienced therapists (2%)
- ■ Everything was harmful (1%)
- ■ Other

35%
12%
7%
7%
5%
4%
4%
4%
2%
1%
20%

Out of 133 responses

Now let's look more deeply at what men who responded to our questionnaire said about some of these less helpful or even harmful efforts.

## Unsupportive, Gay-Affirming, or Inexperienced Therapists

What was less helpful, or even harmful?

- "I went to a therapist who did not believe in change and did not respect my decision to change. He wanted me to live a gay life. After four sessions, I left him."

  — Jose, 26, Mexico, page 78

- "When I was told it was a choice. When I was told that I would never be able to change and to find a way to deal with it. When therapist after therapist did not know anything about helping someone with SSA."

  — Jeddy, 29, Texas, page 53

- "My psychologist saying that I would not be able to live in a heterosexual marriage without having a male lover in addition."

  — "Gunnar," Norway

- "One therapist I saw told me that I was gay and that I should come out of the closet. I was offended and never went back to see him again. If only I could tell him how wrong he was."

  — Steve, 55, Florida, page 103

*The pie charts in this book present a profile of those who responded to the People Can Change questionnaire from which the 54 brief summaries were drawn. They do not indicate representative samplings of SSA or gay populations or of all those who have attempted sexual-orientation changes.*

- "Therapists who had no business trying to help me. Some had no respect for my therapeutic goals, i.e., reduction of SSA feelings and increase in OSA feelings."

  — Blake, 59, California, page 91

- "Gay-affirming therapy was extremely harmful and disempowering. The entire process of pro-gay therapy (as I experienced it in groups and in church settings) was designed to reduce 'who I was' to a very small and convenient sexual identity and then to blame all of my life's problems and unresolved feelings on society's unwillingness to accept that 'type.'

  "I know some people who even contemplated suicide because gay-affirming groups, movements and therapists convinced them they had no power of discernment over their sexual orientation and could make no choices about how they would feel, live or form relationships if such choices even questioned 'gayness' in any way. I found gay-affirming therapy to be extremely fraudulent and misleading because it promised a fulfillment, wholeness and peace that never came."

  — C.D., 41, Massachusetts, page 105

- "My experiences with a therapist who told me I was born gay were, in my opinion, harmful. I would go to this therapist with relative peace of mind, not even planning on doing work related to my same-sex attractions. He kept steering the conversation to same-sex attractions. I would leave incredibly agitated, feeling like I hadn't been heard. He simply wrote off the parts of my experiences that could not be explained in the scenario he was trying to convince me of: that people are born gay and there was nothing that could change sexual attractions. This was after I had already experienced some changes in my attractions. He taught me just how damaging it can be when a therapist pushes an agenda onto his client. It was as if I didn't matter as a person."

  — Benjamin, 37, California, page 93

## Unsupportive, Gay-Affirming Family and Friends

- "From one side, I felt pressure from people telling me that I needed to accept my attractions and embrace them, and from the other side that all I needed to do is pray to God and it will go away. I felt I didn't have the freedom to choose for my own. Both kept me from clearly understanding what this actually means and what could help me to become the man I really wanted to be."

  — Stephan, 34, Germany, page 58

- "Well-meaning friends and family who told me to 'just stop.'"

  — Robert, 47, Texas, page 76

- "I frequently encountered, and still do, people who told me that what I was trying to accomplish was impossible, unhealthy, and foolish. These people did not know me. They did not take time to learn about me. They did not care about me. However, this did not stop them from attempting to discourage or dissuade me from attempting to live my life. This alienated me even more from people and led to intense despair. I am lucky that organizations like People Can Change and North Star International existed and helped me learn that other people had in fact been successful in this endeavor."

  — Kevin, 29, Idaho, page 49

# Inexperienced or Less Supportive Pastoral Counselors

- "The most harmful thing was when I would stumble and my pastors would criticize me for it or say that I had not repented. That just made me depressed and more tempted to SSA. Or if I said I was struggling or confessed some sin and they just didn't respond. Or if they thought I should not talk to young men in my church because I would be attracted to them. In fact, it was when I was talking to them and acting like a peer with all the men that I felt the *least* SSA."

  — "Clark," 39, Indiana

- "Having the pastor who was counseling me hint that my progress was so slow that we might stop meeting. Feeling rejection even from him."

  — Scott, 51, Iowa, page 52

# 'All of It Was Harmful'

Two men who responded to the questionnaire reported that everything they tried was harmful, suggesting that they regretted the attempt overall.

- "It was harmful to start with the premise that I was broken and needed to be fixed. That increased my angst and depression and led me to suicidal thoughts. The process itself wasn't bad but the eventual goal of reducing my SSA was."

  — "Tom," 35, Colorado

- "Any and all change therapy or reparative therapy [was harmful]. Church groups and ministries, experiential workshops/retreats, were all harmful as I experienced a LARGE amount of shame, guilt, and hopelessness as I could not change my orientation or lessen my attraction toward my same sex no matter how hard I tried, even without having ever acted out sexually."

  — "Brad," 30, Tennessee

These two responses were quite rare. Presumably, however, People Can Change would have received more such responses had we sought to find and survey an unbiased, representative sample of everyone who had every participated in sexual-orientation change programs. Remember that People Can Change sent the questionnaire out to our own data base of past, current and potential future participants in our programs. And we specifically said we were looking for "personal accounts demonstrating that, yes, some people really have reduced or eliminated their same-sex attractions through deliberate interventions like counseling, experiential weekend programs, non-sexual same-gender bonding, etc."

From the qualitative information we collected, there is no way to determine how prevalent negative reactions to sexual-orientation change efforts might be. These two anecdotal responses give us a sense of what those who feel harmed by these efforts might experience—and with that awareness should come empathy and compassion. It's unfortunate, certainly. Even tragic, perhaps. But that reaction must be balanced with the reality that a great many others do benefit enormously from the same programs and essentially the same efforts.

# 'None of It Was Harmful'; It Was Life-Saving

Contrast this with the numerous men who said the opposite—that *nothing* they experienced in their change efforts was harmful. On the contrary, it was life-saving for many. Of the 50-plus men profiled here, 16 reported that they had suicidal thoughts or even attempted suicide before they began their sexual-orientation change efforts. Their commitment to understanding and resolving the underlying causes and unmet needs driving their same-sex attractions literally saved their lives.

- "There have been no harmful effects from my efforts. In fact, it is only the opposite that has occurred. I was depressed and suicidal before this work."

    — Steve, 55, Florida, page 103

- "I often had thoughts of suicide and depression before seeking to understand and change my attractions. I have NEVER had a suicidal thought since beginning that process. This journey to greater awareness and authenticity has been like stepping from a dark grave into the light of day and fresh air!"

    — "Richard," 45, Oregon, page 73

- "I was so conflicted before my change efforts, that I became seriously suicidal. Attempting to live and embrace a homosexual lifestyle was very damaging to me. Since learning that change is possible, and beginning my own personal journey, I have experienced increasing peace of mind, improved self-esteem, and no suicidal thoughts."

    —Robert, 47, Texas, page 76

- "I can honestly say that the Journey Into Manhood weekend has helped me save my marriage and even my life. It has put me on a path of healing. My entire experience has been a positive one. I no longer feel despair and hopeless like before. I no longer think of suicide as an option. I know I would not be happy living a gay life. Although the journey of healing has not been an easy one, it has been the best decision for me. I am happier, more confident, and enjoying life now than I ever did before."

    — "Jerry," 43, Maryland, page 102

- "I was suicidal when I was in that life style, but after I got out of it I have found that I am happier and more relaxed in my life."

    — Samuel, 38, South Africa, page 68

Perhaps Jeremy said it best when he commented:

- "I cannot imagine how any aspect of sexual-orientation change efforts (SOCE) could be harmful. Every aspect of reparative therapy and all of the SOCE programs are aimed at improving self-esteem and self-acceptance. That is the primary basis of them all. I have seen such an improvement in my self-esteem and confidence that I would have to say all of the SOCE has been worth it—and would still be worth it even if I hadn't experienced any change in my sexual orientation. In fact, the benefits to my emotional health are even more important than the benefits of reduced same-sex attraction."

    — Jeremy, 36, Texas, page 39

# How My Sexual Attractions Have Changed

We don't need anyone to prove to us that sexual-orientation change is possible. We know firsthand that it is—at least to some degree, and at least for some people—because we've experienced it ourselves. We know it because we've lived it.

Now a very brief profile of who we are.

The 54 first-person accounts that follow have been selected, somewhat randomly, from responses that 173 men submitted to a People Can Change questionnaire in late 2013. Of those 173 men:

- Respondents range in age from 22 to 69, with an average age of 41.

- Four out of five live in the United States.

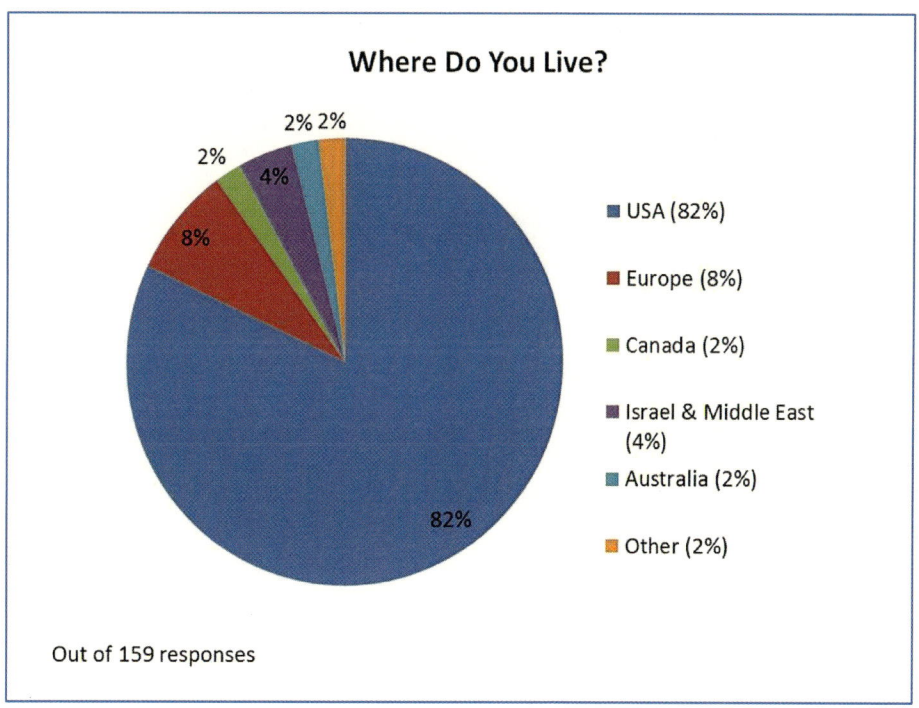

**Where Do You Live?**

- USA (82%)
- Europe (8%)
- Canada (2%)
- Israel & Middle East (4%)
- Australia (2%)
- Other (2%)

2% 2%
2%
4%
8%
82%

Out of 159 responses

*The pie charts in this book present a __profile__ of those who responded to the People Can Change questionnaire from which the 54 brief summaries were drawn. They do not indicate representative samplings of SSA or gay populations or of all those who have attempted sexual-orientation changes.*

- Half are single, 42% are married, and the rest are divorced, widowed, or engaged to marry.

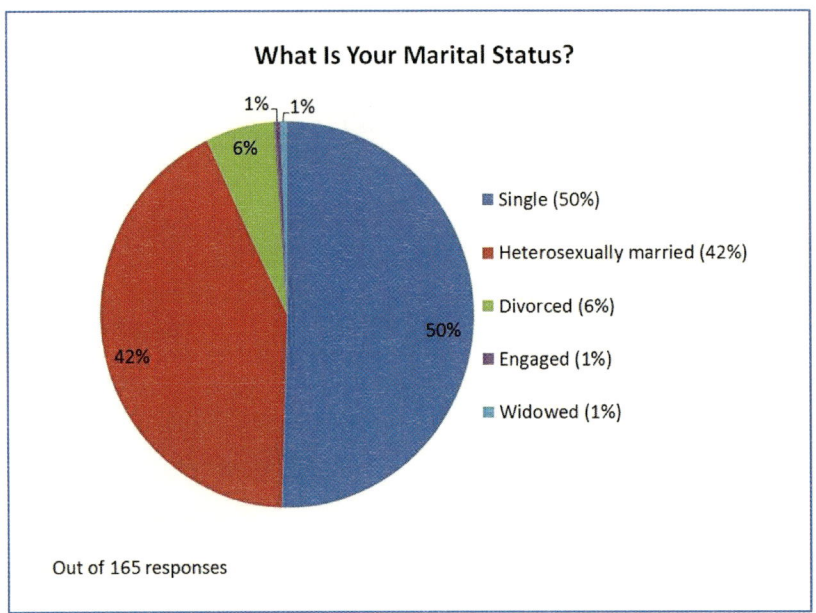

- Four out of five are Christian (Protestant, Catholic, Latter-day Saint or other), 10% are Jewish, 5% are Muslim, and the rest are non-religious.

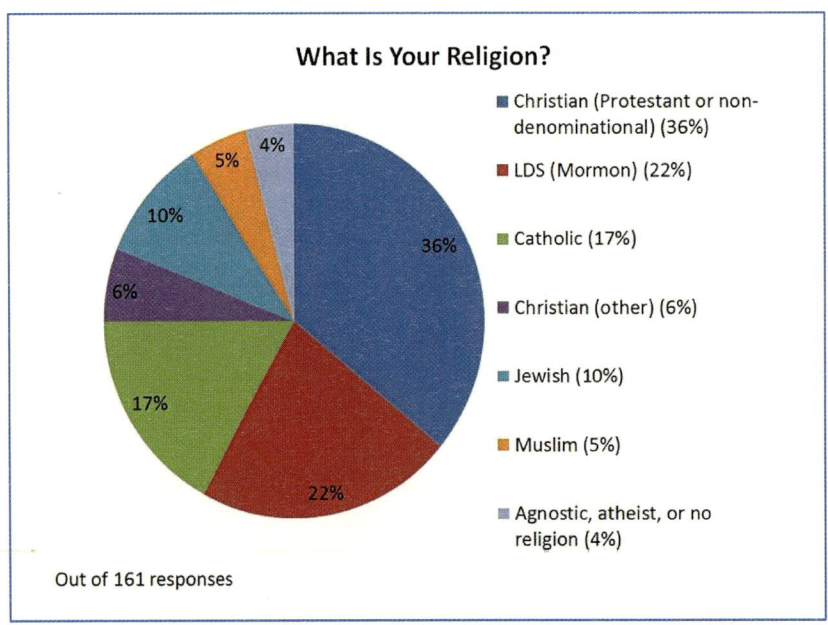

But the one thing we all have in common is that, to one degree or another, and in one way or another, we have experienced change.

Change in our sexual attractions, in most cases, yes. But more important, an increase in peace. A greater sense of wholeness. Of emotional, non-sexual connection to the masculine—our own masculinity and to the greater world of men. A greater sense of brotherhood, and brotherly love. A moderation or elimination of discordant, unwanted sexual behaviors.

Now here are our stories, from our own authentic experience, in our own words.

# Jeremy, 36, lives in Texas USA, Single, Catholic

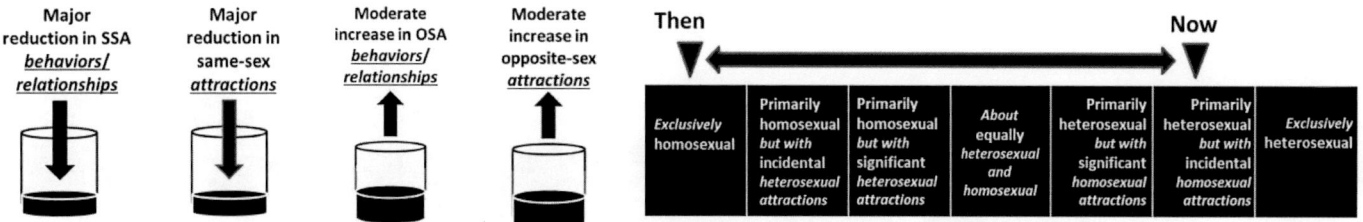

| | | | | Then | | | | | Now | | |
|---|---|---|---|---|---|---|---|---|---|---|---|
| Major reduction in SSA *behaviors/ relationships* | Major reduction in same-sex *attractions* | Moderate increase in OSA *behaviors/ relationships* | Moderate increase in opposite-sex *attractions* | | Exclusively homosexual | Primarily homosexual *but with incidental heterosexual attractions* | Primarily homosexual *but with significant heterosexual attractions* | About equally *heterosexual and* homosexual | Primarily heterosexual *but with significant homosexual attractions* | Primarily heterosexual *but with incidental homosexual attractions* | Exclusively heterosexual |

**SSA "then"**

I began identifying myself as gay when I was in junior high school. I began pursuing gay relationships when I was in high school and continued through several gay relationships throughout my 20s. I did not experience any opposite-sex attraction during those years. I participated in several gay pride parades and had a live-in partner for two years. I used to have sex with other men several times a week. I was completely addicted to homosexual behavior and I viewed every man I met in terms of his physical appearance. Even though my orientation was completely toward my own gender, I never really felt happy with the way my life was going. I didn't feel that that life was compatible with my faith, and over time I realized I couldn't ignore my conscience any longer.

**Motivations**

I eventually came to the conclusion that gay relationships were never going to be fulfilling for me, and I wanted to find another alternative.

**SSA now**

In late 2009, I began pursuing reparative therapy—at first with minimal expectations. I knew it would be beneficial for emotional healing, but was unsure if anyone could help me with the SSA. Through reparative therapy I have experienced a significant decrease in my SSA. I have also experienced major healing for emotional wounds and have seen every aspect of my life improve over the last three years. Now, my SSA is extremely rare. I have not acted out with another man in over three years and do not have the desire to pursue men sexually or to view pornography. My SSA is limited to random thoughts a few times a month, but those are much less controlling or influential on my life.

**What brought about change?**

I worked with Dr. Joseph Nicolosi Jr. in reparative therapy for about two years (weekly) from late 2009 through the end of 2011. This included EMDR therapy for addressing trauma at the roots of my sexual addiction. I also attended the Journey Into Manhood weekend and participated in several follow-up reunions and retreats. I currently lead a small support group that I started which has helped me and many others to continue to grow emotionally and spiritually. The therapy and experiential weekends helped more than I could have ever imagined. Every aspect of my life is better today, and I'm extremely grateful.

**Most helpful?**

Journey Into Manhood, reparative therapy with Dr. Joseph Nicolosi, Junior. Life coaching with individuals from JONAH and People Can Change.

**Less helpful, or even harmful?**

I cannot imagine how any aspect of sexual-orientation change efforts (SOCE) could be harmful. Every aspect of reparative therapy and all of the SOCE programs are aimed at improving self-esteem and self-acceptance. That is the primary basis of them all. I have seen such an improvement in my self-esteem and confidence that I would have to say all of the SOCE has been worth it—and would still be worth it even if I hadn't experienced any change in my sexual orientation. In fact, the benefits to my emotional health are even more important than the benefits of reduced same-sex attraction.

**Any other benefits?**

Yes, I have seen every aspect of my life improve. I feel a lot more assertive and confident at work and in all of my personal relationships. This has made me a much more effective leader and enabled me to be much more effective in my relationships with family and friends. Everyone has noticed a major improvement. I am happier than I've ever been.

# Yeshaya, 23, lives in New York USA, Single, Jewish

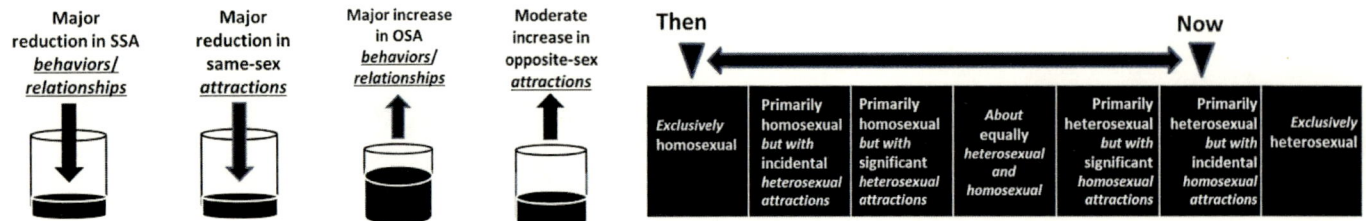

| | | | | | | |
|---|---|---|---|---|---|---|
| Exclusively homosexual | Primarily homosexual but with incidental heterosexual attractions | Primarily homosexual but with significant heterosexual attractions | About equally heterosexual and homosexual | Primarily heterosexual but with significant homosexual attractions | Primarily heterosexual but with incidental homosexual attractions | Exclusively heterosexual |

**SSA "then"**

I was exclusively attracted to men, but the extent of my activity was watching gay porn and masturbating to it. I also had occasional gay fantasies. I did not self-identify as gay, though I was fully conscious of being solely attracted to males. I was not publicly out. I was living a very closeted life. I didn't tell anyone, and no one claimed to know. I had times when I felt very sad and cried about my lot and felt angry about it. But mostly I didn't feel anything at all. I was resigned to the "fact" that there was nothing for me in the future but a single life.

**Motivations**

What motivated me to shift my sexual attraction was my faith. I am an orthodox Jewish man, and I was resigned to the "fact" that I would never be married or loved by a wife. In spite of being a rational, "modern" thinker, I won't give up my faith. When I found out about People Can Change and Journey Into Manhood, I was pretty surprised, but I decided to give it a shot. "What the heck do I have to lose?"

**SSA now**

Now my sexual attractions are almost exclusively hetero. I'm still a virgin, but I am very turned on by pretty girls especially when taken by surprise. I have shifted to viewing hetero or lesbian porn or just viewing pics of cute girls. (Although I plan on stopping the porn habit altogether and remaining in the real world). SSA pops up occasionally in the form of jealousy. However the more I live in reality and allow myself to just be with my buddies, and guys in general, the less I experience this.

**What brought about change?**

My biggest breakthrough was internalizing the fact that, for me, same-sex attraction is a symptom of a warped, low self-image. I began to work on improving my self-image, without focusing too much on the actual SSA issue. I found lots of not-so-pretty stuff, like general lack of confidence, living in a protective bubble, and an inability to realize that there are good people out there who care about me. Finally, I learned how to like myself no matter what, to be present, to chill out, and to own myself and my actions. To breathe, listen, be authentic, and enter old and new relationships with a fresh mind. To be kind to myself and to push myself to work hard.

**Most helpful?**

Seeing a life coach or therapist, "guts work" (emotional processing), hanging with friends more. Experiential personal-growth workshops—whether SSA-specific or not. Talking to people about SSA and self-esteem. Being receptive to help, accepting myself with my flaws, and lots and lots of introspection.

**Less helpful, or even harmful?**

Nothing was harmful.

**Other benefits?**

Before I started all this, I lived in a bubble and had a very low self-esteem. I had no feelings. Now I live in reality, I love me, and I feel normal.

# Christopher, 33, lives in Virginia USA, Heterosexually Married, Christian (Evangelical)

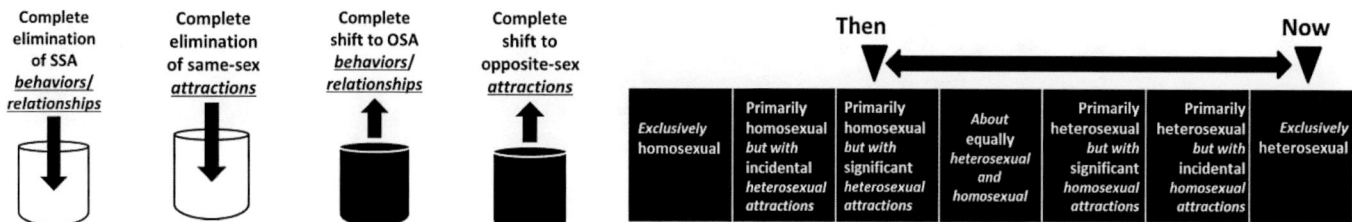

| SSA "then" | At its most challenging point, I felt compelled to have sex with men, not because I wanted to be in a gay relationship, but because I felt inferior and unaccepted by other men. Having sex with men increased my self-esteem temporarily, but left me feeling depressed afterward, because what I really wanted was to feel accepted and loved by men *non-sexually.* |
|---|---|
| **Motivations** | It conflicted with my faith and the belief that I was not born gay. |
| **SSA now** | My SSA is non-existent today. |
| **What brought about change?** | Counseling to deal with sexual abuse, 12 Step support groups, straight friends. When I finally did experience non-sexual love and acceptance from men as a young adult, my need to have sex with men grew less and less desirable and the attractions diminished over time. |
| **Most helpful?** | Non-sexual relationships with straight men. |
| **Less helpful, or even harmful?** | No negative effects, only positive! In fact, it was harmful for me to have sex with men. This question of harm is absurd. We all have the ability to make choices in our lives, including to "act out" or not on behaviors that we feel are immoral. |
| **Any other benefits?** | Every aspect of my life has improved as a result of change. |

# Ali, 25, lives in England, Single (Seeking Marriage), Muslim (Shia)

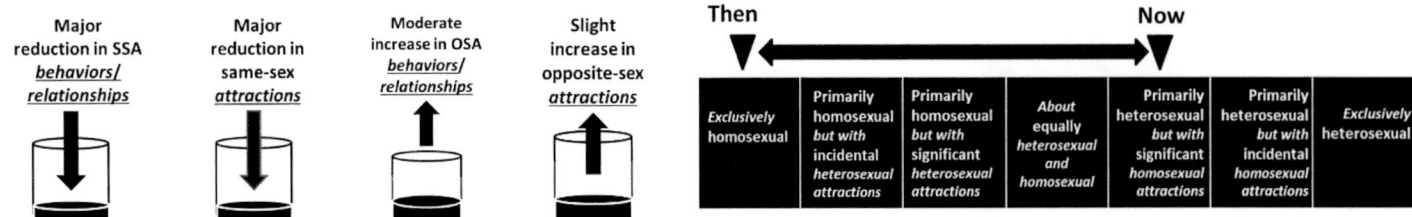

**SSA "then"**

SSA consumed my life. I felt so detached from my own gender and wanted closeness, recognition and affirmation from an older male. I took comfort in porn as an illusory cure. SSA and pornography heavily conflicted with my beliefs, and for a long time I felt as if I was inherently evil and damned to hell. I had an extremely negative view of myself, especially my physical appearance. I hid my SSA for 11 years, until at the age of 23 I suffered moderate clinical depression for two weeks and had to disclose my secret.

**Motivations**

The motivation for me to address my SSA came from me and no one else. I felt that SSA was a developmental flaw in me, as I never understood men or my own gender. The greatest motivation for me was knowing that everyone is given tests, and this *colossal* test was mine. Since God never burdens a soul beyond its capacity (Quran 23:62), I knew I had the strength within me too. I am actually grateful for SSA because without it I wouldn't understand myself or God like I do today.

**SSA now**

I could have never imagined the extent of the change I saw in a short time period. In only a year of self-discovery, my same-sex attractions reduced drastically. This was largely because I now understood what those attractions meant for me and why I had them. In the next year, I felt comfortable to approach the other sex for marriage. I have disclosed my "secret" now to all immediate family members, close friends and even a potential spouse! Now that it has been two years in the journey, SSA is one of the noises in the background. It doesn't consume me anymore. And my latent heterosexuality, which I believe was present all along, has been finally given time to express itself.

**What brought about change?**

Reading Nicolosi's <u>Reparative Therapy for the Male Homosexuality</u> brought tears to my eyes; it was as if it was written about me. These were tears of joy; someone understood me! If I hadn't actively made changes, I would have seen no relief. The best advice I can give is what one therapist gave me: Coming out of SSA is a "lifestyle change." I undertook <u>Bibliotherapy</u>, counseling, retreats, opening the issue to my family and friends, overcoming sport wounds, building friendships, even blogging about my experience and discoveries. I feel like I am discovering myself every day.

**Most helpful?**

<u>Journey Into Manhood</u> was a life-changing experience. I highly value the follow-up <u>video-conference group sessions</u>, as well.

**Less helpful, or even harmful?**

Nothing was harmful.

**Any other benefits?**

I have always been outwardly confident, but not inwardly. These efforts have allowed me to be inwardly confident, accept and love myself, seeing strengths in myself which I couldn't before. I <u>blog</u> in hope of supporting others in the Muslim community, helping people like me.

# Jason, 22, lives in Utah USA, Single, Latter-day Saint

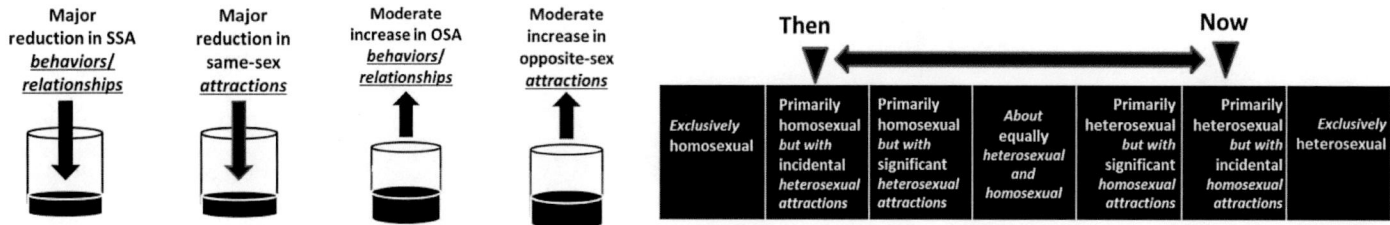

**SSA "then"**

I had an overwhelming addiction to gay pornography and was missing out on a lot of my life because I was so tied to it. I had a brief relationship with one man I met online but it was unsafe and very unhealthy. My true desire is to have an emotional connection with a man—not a sexual one. He was pushing toward the sexual, where I was uninterested and wanted to be celibate.

After ending that relationship, I had another relationship that lasted around six months. I was very attached to him—so much so that I wanted to be with him and give up what I had wanted most of my life. But the relationship was full of heartbreak and ruin. He was physically fixated and didn't want a relationship. I desperately wanted an emotional relationship. After months of depression I took a stand and separated myself completely from him.

I never identified myself as gay throughout my experiences. I felt it would be a commitment to a lifestyle that I truly didn't want to commit to.

**Motivations**

I want a family with a wife and kids of our own. My religious beliefs cause me to see that there is something higher than myself, and if I want to be in line with that, then I should live the way that I believe will make me happy. The way to my happiness is through living in line with my personal beliefs, religion, and the lifestyle that I choose. And I choose not to live a gay lifestyle.

**SSA now**

After taking a stand on the way I wish to live, and sticking to that decision, I have found my attractions to women increasing. My SSA only creeps up on me when I am feeling lonely, but isn't strong enough to cause any harm to the choices I make. After lots of work, my SSA no longer has the intense grip that it once had on me. I do notice attractive women and it delights me that they can take my breath away. I am not sexually active and don't plan to be until after I get married.

I am now living the way that I want and am the happiest I have been in a very long time. I previously kept my struggles to myself but found when I shared my burdens with others they became lighter, and I was able to make the changes I wanted in my life. I found that after letting go of same-sex attractions and determining to live differently, heterosexual feelings began to emerge for me.

**What brought about change?**

My first step was making the personal decision that I wanted to change. Through counseling, I was able to look in towards myself and see the things that were keeping me so fixated on men and wanting to be with them. The personal healing that took place helped to fix and increase the bonds I have with my heterosexual friends. My counselor specialized in helping same-sex-attracted men. He told me he would not force me to change, and that any path I chose he would help me with it. Every counselor should do the same. I let him know the path that I desired, and after a year and a half of sessions, coupled with the amazing weekend programs that I had the privilege of attending, I can say that my same-sex attractions have been greatly diminished and no longer have such a gripping hold on my life. I know I can have and live the life that I choose.

| | |
|---|---|
| **Most helpful?** | <u>Journey Into Manhood</u> and <u>Adventure In Manhood</u> were the two weekends I have experienced. They were incredibly professional, and the brotherhood that was formed at these weekends built up my soul. They also provided me with the tools that I needed to create a better bonding relationship with the men in my life. |
| | Counseling was another major contributor to my personal healing. It provided me with the tools that I needed to help change my everyday life and to make each day a choice—and a happy one even when things are hard. Counseling truly helped me to learn to love myself and solidify the changes I want. |
| | There is also a group that I attend with others who experience SSA, and it has helped me to form connections and healthy bonds with others who are on my same journey. Being friends with people who are trying to live the way you are trying is a wonderful support. |
| **Less helpful, or even harmful?** | Trying to figure out life on my own. |
| **Any other benefits?** | I have increased my relationships with men and women. I have an increase in self-esteem. I truly love my whole self now that I am in line with what I want. I have a greater sense of my personal masculinity. My relationships with my family members have improved. |
| | I am so grateful for all of the resources that were available to me that have helped me to grow personally, spiritually and emotionally. I have learned how to truly love myself and be happy with me and how I choose to live. |

# Tim, 37, lives in Idaho USA, Single, Catholic

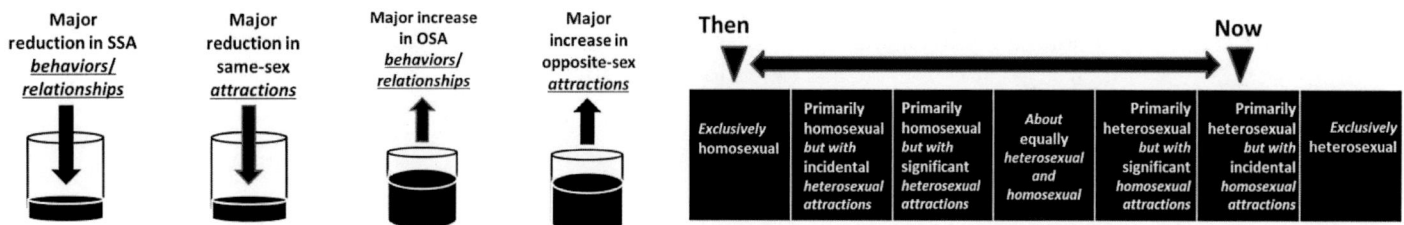

| Major reduction in SSA *behaviors/ relationships* | Major reduction in same-sex *attractions* | Major increase in OSA *behaviors/ relationships* | Major increase in opposite-sex *attractions* | Then ◄─────────────────────────► Now |
|---|---|---|---|---|

| *Exclusively homosexual* | Primarily homosexual *but with incidental heterosexual attractions* | Primarily homosexual *but with significant heterosexual attractions* | *About equally heterosexual and homosexual* | Primarily heterosexual *but with significant homosexual attractions* | Primarily heterosexual *but with incidental homosexual attractions* | *Exclusively heterosexual* |
|---|---|---|---|---|---|---|

**SSA "then"**

Growing up, I was so depressed and had such low self-esteem that I didn't concern myself much with sex or dating at all. I knew I was attracted to men, and I became addicted to porn early on, but until my first sexual experience at age 18, I didn't think much about homosexuality. That first experience was with a man in an adult bookstore. I hated it; I felt disgusting, but I wanted more. For the next five years, I had a serious alcohol problem and contemplated suicide constantly. I was constantly in gay chat rooms, and about twice a month I met up with someone for anonymous sex.

I experimented with being "out" to a few select people, and all of them accepted and encouraged me. I even felt confident that my family would be okay with me being gay. But it still wasn't working. No matter how much sex I had or how many chat rooms I was in, something just didn't feel right, and I still needed more. I drank more and more and started making a plan to live on the streets in Chicago as a male prostitute. I figured it would mean I would take street drugs and be dead before age 25—and I was fine with that.

**Motivations**

I felt like I had been born a homosexual and that something that felt so natural couldn't be wrong. Yet, when I imagined my best fantasy—I'm out and proud, everyone loves me, and I live happily ever after with the man of my dreams—it somehow felt like a consolation prize. Around age 23, I became convinced that all the teachings of the Catholic Church are true and that there was a life out there for me better than I can possibly imagine. Homosexuality was already not working for me, but now it conflicted with my conviction that homosexual acts are immoral. I thought I had only two options and both of them were bad: I either live in incongruity with my world view and give in to my homosexual impulses, or I repress my homosexual impulses and increase my shame and self-hatred. Convinced that I would one day live a life of peace and happiness, I sought a third option.

**SSA now**

Now I identify as completely heterosexual. It has been over 14 years since I've had any sexual behavior with other men and at least 10 years since I've even wanted to. My desire for a homosexual romantic relationship is completely gone, and instead I want to have an intimate, loving , romantic relationship and a lifelong commitment with a woman who is open to children. I already have intimate, loving relationships with men, but they aren't romantic or sexual. They aren't the same thing that I want with one woman. I continue to have an addiction to lust, and the lust is still toward men. I have no desire to change one lust for another and lust after women. My sexual attractions to women are pure and genuine. As I continue my growth toward wholeness, lust will not be a part of my life for either gender.

**What brought about change?**

I had some reparative therapy but mostly I went on experiential weekends like Journey Into Manhood, Adventure In Manhood, Journey Beyond and the New Warrior Training Adventure and applied the principles I learned. This saved and changed my life. I decided to challenge my belief that I was some sort of third gender and didn't belong among the men. I started doing activities with other men that I had always wanted to do but hadn't because I thought I didn't belong. I realized that my homosexual desires were pointing to what I really wanted and needed—authentic connection with other men. I began to nourish authentic male friendships in my everyday life.

| | |
|---|---|
| **Most helpful?** | Realizing that first I had to accept myself just the way I was. Then realizing that nothing was wrong with me because of my homosexual attractions. I wasn't "born that way." The same-sex attractions came about because I didn't feel like I belonged in the world of men, and because I saw women as smothering, selfish, and needy. Then I was able to work on changing those beliefs instead of focusing on the homosexual attractions. |
| | Also, I realized that heterosexuality was not the goal—wholeness was. Like blood from an open wound, my homosexual attractions were only pointing me to where the wound was. Trying to "fix" the homosexual attractions was like only trying to stop the bleeding without ever healing the wound. True healing and wholeness became the goal. |
| | I knew I was wounded because I felt worthless, incapable, and unlovable. I worked at healing these actual wounds without being concerned if my homosexual attractions changed or diminished or not. And the more I did, the more the homosexual attractions diminished without me even trying. |
| **Less helpful, or even harmful?** | When I first started this, I believed that I had to change the homosexual attractions in order to be good or to be accepted. I was motivated primarily by shame, and that did not work. Real change did not begin for me until I learned to receive love (love myself) with all my homosexual attractions, even if they never changed. |
| **Any other benefits?** | By challenging my beliefs about my homosexual desires, I have learned to challenge self-limiting beliefs in other areas of my life. Now I'm doing and accomplishing things I never thought possible before. |

# Sam, 26, lives in Utah USA, Single, Latter-day Saint

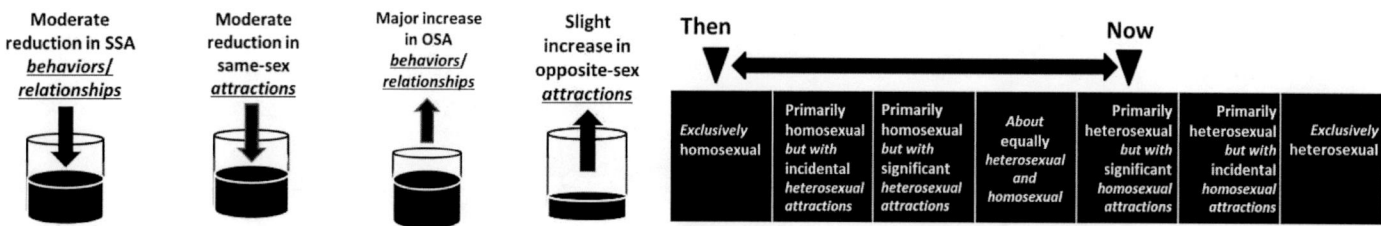

| | | |
|---|---|---|
| **SSA "then"** | Before I started working on my SSA, I felt alone and isolated. I was addicted to same-sex pornography and I knew that was just the beginning. I identified myself as someone who had SSA and I didn't think change was possible. I was extremely unhappy with myself and was even suicidal at times. | |
| **Motivations** | I desire to marry a woman and have a family. When I have acted on homosexual attractions, it has always left me with a bad feeling afterward. My religion is a key factor as well for my motivation. | |
| **SSA now** | I am no longer acting out on my pornography addiction, and this has greatly helped me and my desires. Today, my SSA feelings are significantly less than they were before. Now, when they come up, I can deal with them in healthy ways and in ways that make me feel good about myself afterward. Now, I am starting to lust after women, which never would have happened before. | |
| | I am a 26-year-old male, so reduction of anything sexual is difficult. However, the feelings are more manageable to me, just as I had hoped. There is a sexual attraction to women that was not there before. | |
| **What brought about change?** | I have changed my attitude to reflect that I am a person of worth and these feelings don't control me. I control me. I have done extensive counseling, experiential retreats, and <u>12 Step programs</u>. Without any of these, I know I would not be in the same place I am today. I still have some growing to do, but I like the place I am in now better than before I started working on these feelings. | |
| **Most helpful?** | The most beneficial things to me were the programs through <u>People Can Change</u>. This really helped to kick start everything and push me in the direction I had wanted to go my whole life. | |
| **Less helpful, or even harmful?** | Nothing comes to mind | |
| **Any other benefits?** | I feel more confident and feel comfortable with myself. I feel like I am a man of worth, which wasn't always there before. I feel like my relationships with other men are closer to what I always desired, but they are not sexual like my feelings always told me they had to be. I also feel masculine and a real man for the first time in my life. | |

# Dennis, 54, lives in Texas, Heterosexually Married, Christian

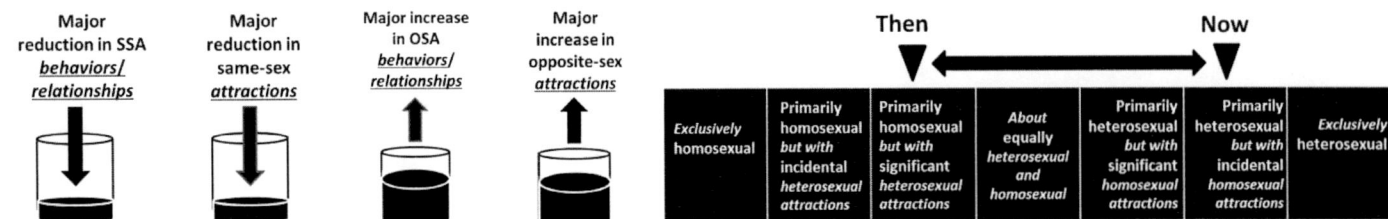

| | Major reduction in SSA *behaviors/ relationships* | Major reduction in same-sex *attractions* | Major increase in OSA *behaviors/ relationships* | Major increase in opposite-sex *attractions* | | Then | | | | Now | |

**SSA "then"**

Prior to recovery, my struggle with SSA was very addictive and out of control. I was compulsively addicted to male pornography and masturbation. Prior to marriage, I also struggled with anonymous sexual encounters at adult video stores.

**Motivations**

As a follower of Jesus Christ, I believe the Bible and believe homosexual behavior is wrong. It is in direct conflict with my beliefs and values as a Christian man. I am married to my wife of 25 years and we have had three great children together. I have never considered myself gay and never will. My same-sex attractions are unwanted, and I have pursued every avenue to change them.

**SSA now**

My SSA is bothersome but not life-dominating. I no longer struggle with pornography or masturbation and have developed good, healthy (non-sexual) relationships with men at large. I struggle with SSA when I am feeling hungry, angry, lonely, tired or disconnected. However, once I deal with the root cause, it goes away.

**What brought about change**

Changes were brought about by:

1. Recovery and accountability groups.
2. Celebrate Recovery and its 12 step program.
3. Reparative Therapy for five-plus years.
4. Experiential retreat: Journey into Manhood.
5. Bibliotherapy: Lots of reading of many books on the subject.

Recovery groups, accountability groups, reparative therapy and experiential weekends have all been crucial in helping me decrease same-sex sexual behaviors. Reparative therapy helped me tremendously in reducing my unwanted same-sex attractions.

**Most helpful**

My accountability and recovery group was the most helpful. This group was primarily comprised of guys who do not struggle with SSA. The Journey into Manhood experiential weekend helped me grow in my masculinity and thereby drastically improved my relationship with my wife, including my sexual relationship with her. My counseling and reparative therapy work helped me tremendously in reducing my unwanted same-sex attractions. My relationship with God was also crucial.

**Less helpful, or even harmful**

Nothing really. Everything I have pursued has helped. I can think of no negative effects resulting from my sexual-orientation change efforts.

**Other benefits?**

Yes, I have grown in my self-awareness and in my identity as a man and follower of Jesus Christ.

**Final comments?**

Change takes time and is an on-going process. The change I have experienced is real and has taken a variety of things to make it happen.

# Kevin, 29, lives in Idaho USA, Heterosexually Married, Latter-day Saint

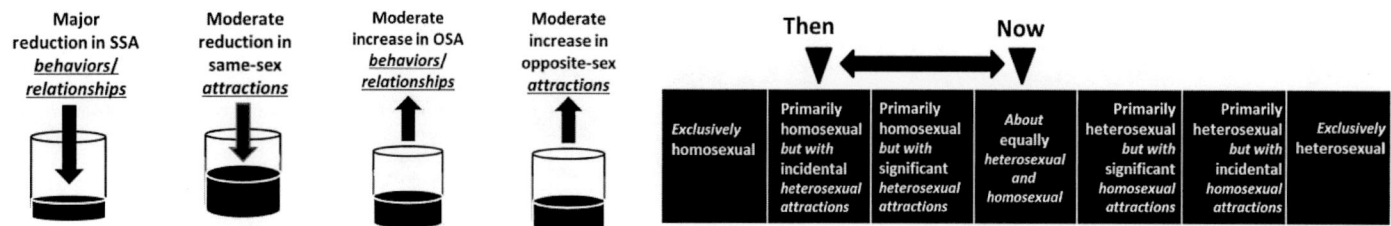

**SSA "then"**

Prior to seeking help, I was in agonizing turmoil. I had denied or repressed my sexuality so much that I did not acknowledge it until after I was married. After coming out to her, I began exploring romantic and sexual relationships with other men without her knowledge. I began to identify as gay, and our sex life virtually ended. The inner conflict became so severe that I was often suicidal—and attempted once. I didn't want to end the marriage; I loved my wife and wanted to raise children with her. However, I knew that I could not handle the stress of maintaining a double-life, and that our relationship would not survive an "open marriage" arrangement.

**Motivations**

I was committed to maintaining my marriage and living in harmony with my personal values. I wanted to reduce the tension between my homosexual attractions and these goals. I believed that by working to reduce the intensity of my homosexual attractions, I would be able to live my life with less stress and depression.

**SSA now**

Today, I have been out of active change efforts for over four years. I continue to be satisfied and fulfilled in my marriage. I no longer experience shame or guilt around my homosexual attractions. I do not experience any conflict between my attractions and my personal value system. I do not feel sexually repressed or incomplete because I am not actively expressing my homosexuality. I believe I am in a situation equal to any individual who is in a committed relationship with one individual and yet still experiences attractions to other individuals. I have learned that when I regularly meet my needs for positive, non-sexual male intimacy, the intensity of my SSA is significantly reduced. I am much more comfortable in my relationship with my wife, and my desire to remain in my marriage has significantly increased. I have been able to increase my fulfillment and satisfaction in my marriage, including in our sexual intimacy.

**What brought about change?**

Primarily by learning to reject messages of shame and inadequacy. My therapist was a major help with this, although we did not work specifically on reducing my homosexuality. I also attended the People Can Change experiential weekend Journey Into Manhood. I found it to be a powerful tool in reducing the shame and isolation I felt. The idea that same-sex attractions stem from incongruence with gender-identity and gender-affiliation did not pathologize or stigmatize those attractions. Instead they normalized them and provided a framework for understanding them in a way that facilitated a successful resolution of my inner conflict.

**Most helpful?**

Individual counseling with a licensed mental health professional who was open to my choices. He was non-judgmental and would have supported me in whatever choice I made. The next most important thing was connection and positive association with other men in situations similar to mine. This was largely accomplished through the People Can Change organization.

# "David," 52, lives in Israel, Heterosexually Married, Jewish

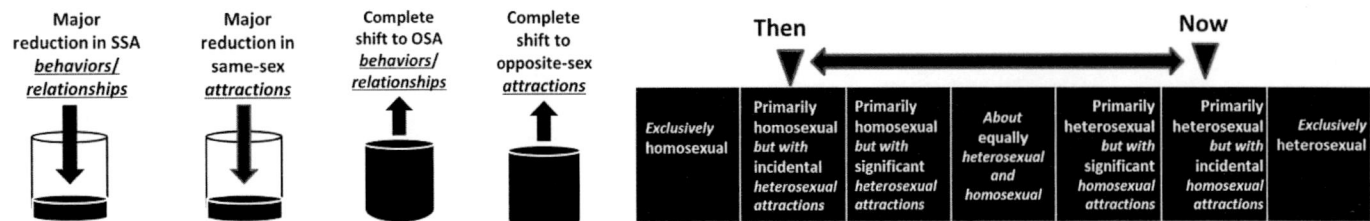

**SSA "then"**    I grew up in the New York metro area, and started going to gay movie houses and other "cruising" venues during high school. I was very sexually active, and enjoyed the attention that the gay world lavishes on young men. However, my emotional life was a series of "crushes" in which I was obsessed with and dependent on father or "bad boy" figures, and then felt devastated when they betrayed me. Being in the gay life in Manhattan generated a rush of excitement that I initially mistook for self-fulfillment. But the lifestyle and my behavior were still driven by my deep insecurity and emotional neediness. I was easily manipulated, and when the rush of an "encounter" wore off, I felt lonely and bad about myself.

I made several attempts during high school and college to find a therapist who could help me, but there were no organizations to help people like me. I stumbled into marriage without significant insight into my SSA, and only later made contact with organizations like JONAH and the National Association for Research and Therapy of Homosexuality (NARTH) that gave me honest information and hope, and pointed me toward therapists and support groups that helped me identify and heal the underlying wounds in my masculine identity. My life has improved greatly as a result!

**Motivations**    Deep dissatisfaction with the gay lifestyle, and a desire to live a physically and emotionally healthier life. Deep conflict between the homosexual agenda—and how the homosexual lifestyle actually plays out—and my personal values and religious beliefs. Desire for a healthy family life based on trust, love, and commitment—which despite media imagery I did not see in the gay community.

**SSA now**    I am now happily married with children. I have not had any physical contact with another man for over 10 years. My lived sexuality is overwhelmingly heterosexual. When I am depressed, or feeling emotional distress, gay imagery or feelings of inferiority and neediness towards other men appear. But I know this is just the old "non-solution" presenting itself.

**What brought about change?**
1. Reached out to the JONAH organization, joined their support group, and started reading background materials on their website.

2. Reached out to NARTH and other sources of information.

3. Persevered with therapy for several years, to uncover and finally heal childhood family patterns and traumatic experiences that contributed to my SSA.

4. Reached out to my local clergy and community about my depression and isolation.

5. Attended men's growth weekends—both for general and SSA populations—recommended by JONAH. The most powerful of these was Journey Into Manhood sponsored by the People Can Change organization. These weekends introduced me to "guts work"—physical work to release and express emotional wounds—and to practical reality-check and problem-solving skills. They also gave me a support group of fellow men.

6. Joined a 12-step group for online porn addicts, while continuing with the support groups of JONAH and the men's weekends.

I currently attend a weekly SSA support group, and a daily phone call with the 12-step porn addiction group—in addition to regular "check-in" calls with the friends I have made in these groups.

| | |
|---|---|
| **Most helpful?** | Long-term dialogue in JONAH support groups. Weekends and support groups of People Can Change and support groups of Call of the Shofar. |
| **Less helpful, or even harmful?** | Lots of misinformation about how normal and healthy homosexuality was—which was directly contradictory to my personal observation and experience! People implying I was a failure for not making the gay life work—or somehow a "traitor to the cause" for not accepting the unsatisfactory gay lifestyle. |
| | NOTHING I experienced in my healing process approaches the dysfunctional, manipulative, and exploitative behaviors that I encountered in gay Manhattan. |
| | The work can be difficult. It can involve probing the most painful parts of one's personal history, and confronting one's deepest fears. This can make this therapy especially difficult for those with very brittle self-worth. The work often involves exposing yourself to groups of men—and this can be very challenging to men who feel deeply inferior, or who feel they have been rejected by men in the past. So it's easier to push away the therapy, and preserve what little sense of self one has. I understand where these people are coming from—and feel compassion for them. But the therapy works—and is not damaging at all. In fact, most of the techniques I've worked with are the same tools used for compulsive behaviors (such as 12-step programs and emotional work). |
| **Any other benefits?** | I definitely feel more positive and confident about myself as a person. I am more secure in the knowledge that I am worthy and equal to others—which makes me more open to REAL friendships and closeness with men, which is what I really always craved. I am very grateful to my wife for standing by me—which has been a great source of self-esteem. I am grateful to have become a father—I found out how much I had to give, stopped feeling needy and started feeling blessed, and "grew up" in many ways. |
| **Final comment?** | Read more about my story – and my responses to reader's questions – at http://www.aish.com/authors/48868967.html |

# Scott, 51 lives in Iowa USA, Heterosexually Married, Christian (Protestant)

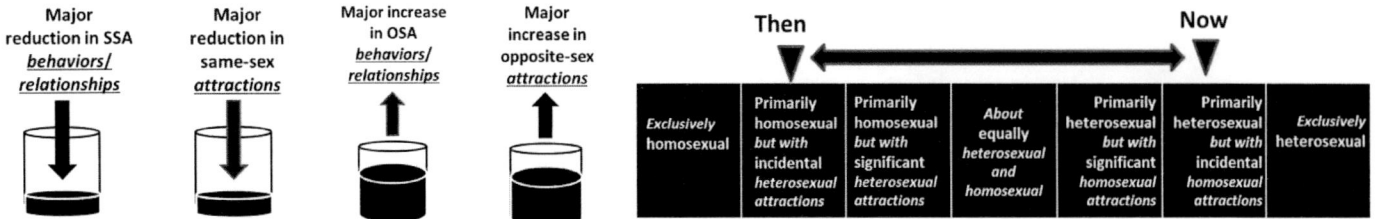

**SSA "then"**

I considered my SSA to be very strong. I was looking at homosexual pornography every chance I had. I was engaged in homosexual fantasy much of the time—and always when I was making love to my wife. I was not engaging in sex with men; I was too afraid and ashamed. However, I decided I was ready to try it—fear and shame be damned. I wanted above all else to seek a man out and have unprotected sex with him. I used to not have desires for women. You may ask, Then why did you marry a woman? The answer is that I did not want to grow old alone. I wanted to have and raise kids. And I wanted to appear "normal."

**Motivations**

My religious beliefs, my wife, and my two young children—pretty much equally.

**SSA now**

My SSA is weaker, much weaker, and seems to be fading as time goes by. The desire is just not there and even fantasy has become primarily heterosexual in nature. This is not a conscious choice, just what I find happening. In bed with my wife, my focus is mainly on her—how much I desire her, how much I love her, how much I want to please her. Sexual relations with her have increased dramatically. At one point I really did not have a sexual desire for her. Now I can't seem to keep my hands off of her. The only times when same-sex sexual feelings, attractions and desires start to creep back into my life are when I feel I am unable to connect with men in a healthy, non-sexual way.

**What brought about change?**

Experiential training/retreats. First was Edge Venture, where I was able to get rid of much of the shame I felt over my SSA desires. Being able to admit my attractions to "straight" men and still be accepted by them was huge for me. Second was Journey into Manhood. My SSA desires decreased dramatically—maybe by half. I thought that this might be temporary, but a year later I would have to say that my desires had dropped even further—maybe by 75%. Third was Journey Beyond. SSA desires are now at about 2% of what they used to be. Since then, counseling and reaching out to men in friendship as an equal have brought about further growth and change.

**Most helpful?**

These last two years, I have attended three men's experiential weekends. It is here that I have seen the greatest results: Being able, in a controlled environment, to interact with men successfully in a non-sexual way; to see that I am like them; I am accepted as one of them; that they hurt like me—whether they are dealing with SSA or not.

**Less helpful, or even harmful?**

Having the pastor who was counseling me hint that my progress was so slow that we might stop meeting. Feeling rejection from even him.

**Any other benefits?**

Emotionally, I am a much healthier person. I used to have really deep emotional lows, to the point that I considered suicide several times. Now, I am happy. I like myself, where before I did not. My self-esteem is much greater than it has ever been. I feel respected and appreciated by men, where before I felt merely tolerated (or downright rejected) by them. My marriage is very strong. I love her more deeply than ever. I feel masculine; before I did not. I feel like an adult; before I felt like an 8-year-old boy stuck in a 48-year-old body of a man.

# Jeddy, 29, lives in Texas USA, Heterosexually Married, Latter-day Saint

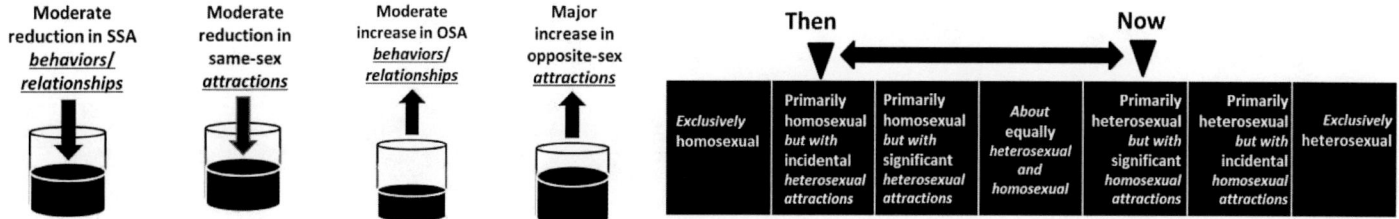

**SSA "then"**

My SSA peaked at my teenage years. I was living a double life. Nobody knew I was attracted to men, not even my molester. I was afraid to tell anyone. I was afraid I would be made fun of, that my church would reject me and my dad would kick me out of the house. I was miserable. The fight going on in my mind every day became unbearable. I couldn't even tell my best friends. I tried having girlfriends, but I was never able to be authentic. I thought they were pretty, but emotionally, I was not there.

**Motivations**

My initial motivation was to become a better husband to my new wife. But then I came to realize my real motivation is that I deserve to be happy, less burdened, more loved and cared for. I deserve to not be chained to what was done to me when I was younger. I also am motivated as a future father. I want to start a new path to a different kind of environment for my future children.

**SSA now**

Today, my SSA is nothing compared to when I was an adolescent. I find my wife and other women beautiful and honor their beauty. I might be attracted to a man, but dismiss the thought as soon as it enters. I know that all I am seeking there is superficial. It has no depth. Whereas with my wife, it is genuine love.

Though I am still attracted to men in the physical since, I no longer wonder what could have been. I don't feel that moving my way towards a heterosexual lifestyle is wrong or a way out. I am comfortable and stronger now. I no longer want to live a double life. My life is my wife, my faith and my journey. Before it was in a constant state of denial and hiding.

**What brought about change?**

People Can Change is what changed my life. It is what started my path out of SSA. It helped me become a better husband, friend, son, brother and son of God. I am able to see reality now instead of hiding in a double life. I am able to accept myself.

It took me a while to find what I needed. I went through a year of finding the right therapist. It helped initially, but then plateaued. When I found reparative therapy through People Can Change, it was an answer to a 17-year prayer. Finally, I wasn't alone. Finally, I was heard and there were people who wanted to help me. It all began to make sense. I hit the ground running and have not stopped since.

**Most helpful?**

People Can Change. Not just stopping with the weekend either. Staffing other weekends, Journey Beyond and men's reunions and groups. I have a whole network of men to depend on for help now.

**Less helpful, or even harmful?**

When I was told it was a choice. When I was told that I would never be able to change and to find a way to deal with it. When therapist after therapist did not know anything about helping someone with SSA.

**Other benefits?**

My marriage, work, family, and friendships have all benefited. I myself am a different person now. I believe in myself. I see hope.

# Mohamed, 34, lives in United Kingdom, Single, Muslim

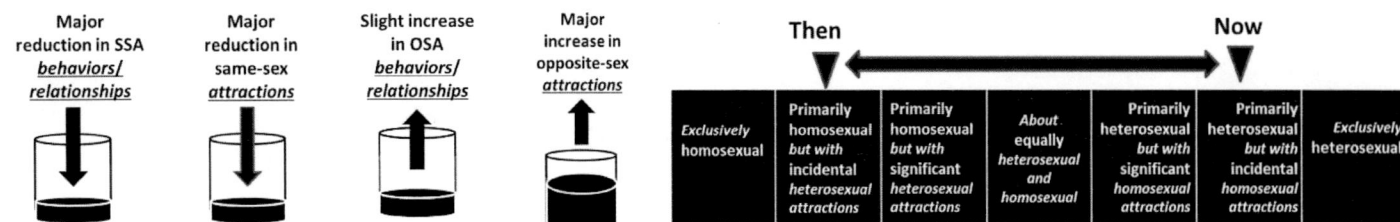

**SSA "then"**

I identified as gay when I was about 19. Previous to that I'd always had a fascination with the same gender, albeit it was never sexualized. At 19, when I was at university, in talking to others it seemed like homosexuality was the only viable way to explain why I was the way I was. Then my behaviors reinforced the homosexual feelings (reward mechanism, Pavlov's dogs, all that sort of stuff) which cemented the feelings. At 21, I realized that my religion was more important than the transient nature of this life, and if God didn't want me to act in a certain way then I accepted His authority over my life.

It was hell though. From about 21 to 27, I didn't engage in same-sex behavior, but I was miserable because in my mind I was still homosexual. I gave up and asked God to show me a way out.

**Motivations**

I felt that I wasn't reaching my potential. I felt that my body was naturally created heterosexual (physically, biologically, endocrinologically) but my psychology wasn't in step. I wanted more from life. Marriage. Children. To reach my fullest potential as a human male.

**SSA now**

I don't have same-sex attractions today in the sense that when I see a good-looking guy I don't want to engage with him in any sort of sexual way. I see him as an equal—a brother with good and bad qualities—just like me. If I see an attractive quality in him, it's because I know I desire that quality in myself.

I have some opposite-sex attractions now. I recognize women as my natural partner. But circumstances at home and within myself still hold me back somewhat from pursuing this—not because of a lack of attraction but perhaps a lack of confidence.

**What brought about change?**

I went on pilgrimage with a group of other brothers and I got the feeling of worthiness and masculinity and brotherhood that I'd always craved. I came back home and started to attend a <u>MANS</u> group frequented by people who had been on <u>People Can Change's Journey Into Manhood</u> weekend. It really helped to understand the psychology of the same-sex attraction, what could practically be done to achieve growth, etc. The knowledge of what underlay the homosexuality in itself was incredibly liberating. At least I knew why, and I knew how to progress.

**Most helpful?**

It was incredibly liberating to come to understand that my attraction to other men at its core wasn't because of homosexuality per se but because of a deeper unmet need for me to connect with masculinity in order to complete my own growth. I realized that interacting with the men in a sexual nature wasn't helping me attain masculinity within myself. It was futile—like drinking salt water to quench a thirst.

Looking into my religion taught me to look objectively at my creation. And everything about my body was heterosexual. Looking into SSA therapy made me realize what I always knew. That it was about wanting to *be* the guy rather than wanting to be *with* him. Going to the <u>MANS</u> group, reading a lot on <u>NARTH</u> and actually making an effort to engage with more heterosexual males has helped me understand my place as a man among men and made me grow into a more comfortable sense of my masculinity.

| | |
|---|---|
| **Less helpful, or even harmful?** | The personalities at the MANS support group sometimes became an issue because all of us were hurt in some way growing up. We all had our individual habits and insecurities and sensitivities. Sometimes that didn't help. I realized I needed to be around men, especially Muslim, heterosexual, confident and masculine men. I respect the other brothers going through SSA therapy. But sometimes they can't help me as much when they still have so many of their own issues to work through. |
| **Any other benefits?** | I don't judge people as quickly. It has taught me empathy. It has brought me closer to God. It has made me a lot more comfortable in my own skin. The self-esteem improvement and the increase in inner masculinity aren't actually benefits as such—they are the *core* to the issue, not some nice side effect. It is the homosexuality in itself that was a side issue for me that got resolved when the self-esteem and the inner masculinity increased. |

# Tim, 48, lives in Oregon USA, Single, Christian (Anglican)

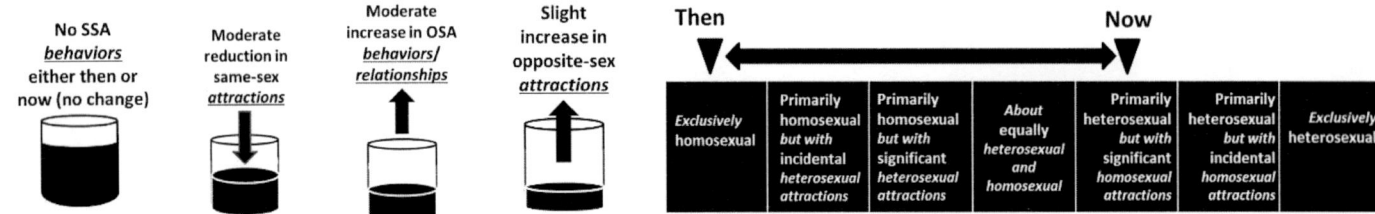

| | | | |
|---|---|---|---|
| **No SSA** *behaviors* either then or now (no change) | **Moderate reduction in** same-sex *attractions* | **Moderate increase in OSA** *behaviors/* *relationships* | **Slight increase in opposite-sex** *attractions* |

| | | | | | | |
|---|---|---|---|---|---|---|
| *Exclusively homosexual* | Primarily homosexual *but with* incidental heterosexual attractions | Primarily homosexual *but with* significant heterosexual attractions | About equally heterosexual and homosexual | Primarily heterosexual *but with* significant homosexual attractions | Primarily heterosexual *but with* incidental homosexual attractions | *Exclusively heterosexual* |

**SSA "then"**

Before I began looking at the roots of my SSA, I *never* felt like "one of the guys" but always felt as if I was more like the women, or like some other entity altogether. I was more comfortable being around women than men, and felt enmeshed with them. My sexual impulses were exclusively for men. I was depressed and suicidal.

**Motivations**

What I saw of the men I knew who had gone into the homosexual lifestyle was unappealing. It seemed to me to be a world of promiscuity, and lacked depth. I was looking for a committed family of men to be in my life, and it seemed to me that I wouldn't necessarily find that level of fidelity in the homosexual community. In addition I didn't see anyone in an openly gay life that I wanted to be like. I wanted to live a life as *man*, not defining myself by whatever my sexual impulses may be.

**SSA now**

Today I feel very grounded in my male identity. My sexual impulses for women are minimal, but relationally I love interacting and partnering with them as people who are at their essence different from who I am. In terms of men, I never acted out before, so that hasn't changed, but now I feel much more on equal grounds with other men.

What I can say with complete confidence is that the locus of my male identity is found within my body, not in the body of another man. I also enjoy immensely the difference between men and women, and relish being a man, and different from the women in my life. Both of these aspects of my life were completely absent before I began critically examining my impulses and behavior.

My core relational needs are still for men, but I have found considerable ways of meeting those needs in non-sexual ways in brotherhood that are completely filling, and lacking nothing. These brothers are family. It is when I am not getting my needs met in healthy, consistent, non-sexual ways that I can find myself beginning to objectify men.

**What brought about change?**

Counseling, groups like People Can Change, supportive men's groups where I could be honest and have men in my life who know everything about me.

**Most helpful?**

Being known and having a safe place to work through things past, present and future, and being in a community that doesn't define an individual based on his or her sexual impulses.

**Less helpful, or even harmful?**

Nothing.

**Any other benefits?**

Certainly, here is where I felt change through the roof. My confidence in who I am as a man, my ability to stand up and speak my truth and be heard, my letting go of defining myself by SSA or anything else, my leadership abilities, care of others, and soundness of mind have grown enormously. I would not be the secure leader and man that I am today if it wasn't for this work.

**Final comment?**

Everyone's journey in this is different to some extent, and one model does not fit all.

# Joseph, 34, lives in Utah USA, Single, Latter-day Saint

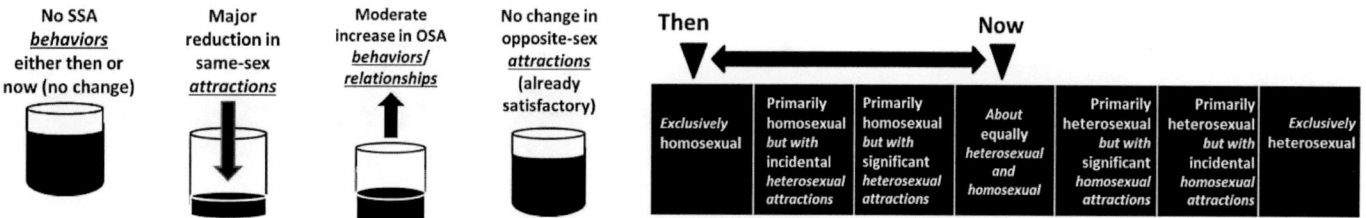

| | | |
|---|---|---|
| **SSA "then"** | My SSA has been hard to deal with my whole life. I had moments that I wanted to "act out" where the feeling was almost painful, but deep down I knew I would regret doing it. I spent years carrying the burden alone and trying to deal with it on my own as I struggled down a path of dating women, which seemed to be an endless and hopeless path. | |
| **Motivations** | I have multiple reasons for wanting to diminish or get rid of my same-sex attractions. First and foremost is what I believe to be right for me. I want a traditional family and want my faith and beliefs to be congruent with my actions. | |
| **SSA now** | Once I started getting help with my unwanted SSA, I have started to feel whole again, and I have gained a brighter hope for my desire to have a family and have even felt a stronger attraction to women. I have never been sexually active. My desire to be sexual with men was becoming increasingly strong. But that has now reduced significantly. | |
| **What brought about change?** | I started meeting with a counselor and attended the Journey Into Manhood weekend. Both have been life-changing and instrumental in my progress. | |
| **Most helpful?** | Attending the Journey Into Manhood and meeting with a therapist. | |
| **Less helpful, or even harmful?** | Nothing | |
| **Any other benefits?** | My relationships with other guys have improved, and my confidence has increased. | |
| **Final comment?** | There are thousands like me who don't want their feelings of SSA, and having a resource or avenue to get help will literally save lives. I have seen people change and seen people come away from these programs with a brighter hope and renewed self-confidence. If one person has a bad experience for some reason, that doesn't mean he should potentially ruin what is considered a godsend to many others. | |

# Stephan, 34, lives in Germany, Heterosexually Married, Latter-day Saint

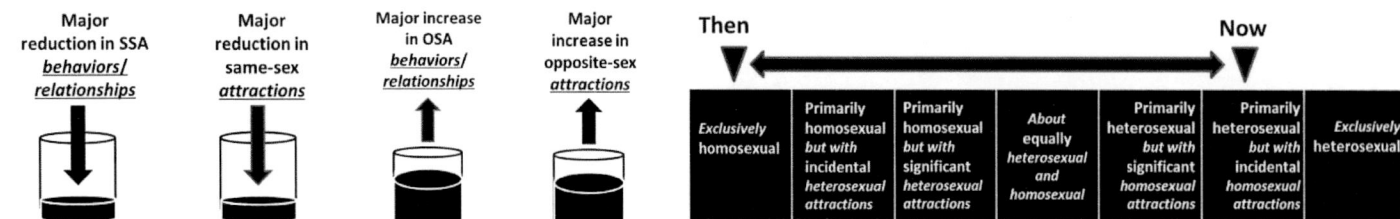

**SSA "then"**

I was exclusively attracted to men, and my attractions were really strong. I wanted closeness and affection from men and tried to get that by being sexually active with them. I identified as gay. I lived a double life of a gay man and a prefect son. I was absolutely unhappy, I felt alone and wasn't able to relate to anybody. I was oftentimes devastated and conflicted about my life. I felt that nobody really knew me because I was too afraid to share with them what was going on within me.

**Motivations**

When I was living a gay life I felt this emptiness in my heart. I didn't know where it was coming from but I realized that I need to change. I realized that what I wanted most in my life was not to feel alone—but contrary to what everyone was telling me, pursuing a gay lifestyle made me feel even more alone. I recognized what I really wanted was to have a family and children—to be a dad.

**SSA now**

I don't feel any same-sex attractions for weeks and I notice my opposite-sex attraction being strong and present. I'm absolutely attracted to my wife and want to be with her and enjoy every moment with her. I haven't been sexually active with guys for over 15 years, and have no desire to do so. My same-sex behaviors and attractions have almost completely diminished. I think the main reason for it is that I learned how to connect with other men. I rarely struggle with pornography but I recognize that it is more an effect of feeling disconnected and alone.

**What brought about change?**

My conversations with my church leaders and parents enabled me to open up and start my journey into a more fulfilling life. My wonderful wife helped me to understand a lot of what was going on inside of me. I attended a Journey Into Manhood weekend, went to therapy, attended an Edge Venture weekend, attended Journey Beyond, attended a MANS group in my area and a 12 Step program.

**Most helpful?**

Most helpful for me was the love, acceptance and open conversations with my wife. But also the experiential weekend retreats from People Can Change made a significant difference. Because of them I was able to truly understand who I am and let go of all the shame and baggage in my life. I was able to understand what happened and how to push through all of it. Attending a local MANS group gave me the platform to grow more. Finally, meeting with a counselor and therapist gave me the tools to push through everything from my past that was still there.

**Less helpful, or even harmful?**

From one side, I felt pressure from people telling me that I needed to accept my attractions and embrace them, and from the other side that all I needed to do is pray to God and it will go away. I felt I didn't have the freedom to choose for my own. Both kept me from clearly understanding what this actually means and what could help me to become the man I really wanted to be.

**Any other benefits?**

My efforts never were to change my sexual orientation but to be happy as the man I am—the man God created me to be. I've seen an increase in my self-esteem and renewed confidence. I have much more joy in my life, and I'm much more "present." That had a direct effect on my family and marriage. I relate to my wife more in my own masculinity. My relationships with other men are better. I stopped doubting my friendships. I recognize my own feminine side in myself, which enables me to embrace the femininity of the women around me, especially my wife. My love for her has increased a lot. I'm more secure and confident as a father too.

# "Rafael," 33, lives in Poland, Heterosexually Married, Not Religious.

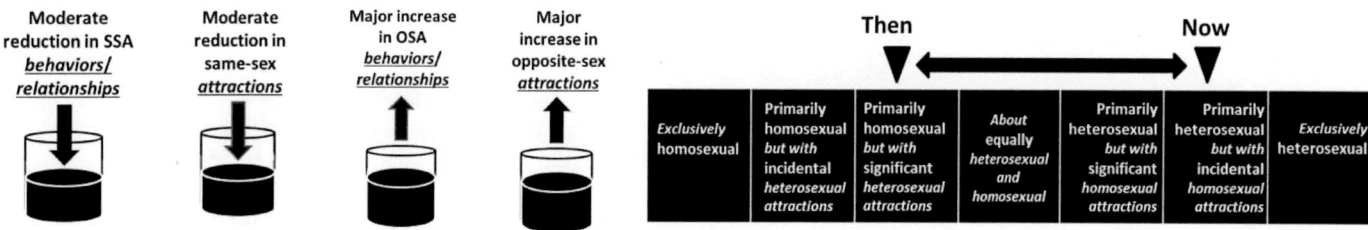

| | | |
|---|---|---|
| **SSA "then"** | I have never identified myself as gay. I just did not know what those desires meant for me and why I was afraid of other men and ashamed to be a man. Today I know the reasons and have resolved them. | |
| **Motivations** | 1. I did not feel it was my real identity. | |
| | 2. I wanted to see what was behind those desires (I never lost my sexual interest in women even though homosexual fantasies appeared). | |
| | 3. I wanted to have children. | |
| **SSA now** | I have a very satisfied sexual life in my heterosexual marriage, although SSA attractions have not diminished totally and they sometimes come back. But I have no "live" sexual actions with other men. | |
| **What brought about change?** | Psychotherapy, 12 Steps (Sexaholics Anonymous), Journey Into Manhood, the New Warrior Training Adventure. | |
| **Most helpful?** | All of them combined. | |
| **Less helpful, or even harmful?** | I haven't experienced any negative effects here. | |
| **Any other benefits?** | Inner sense of masculinity + serenity + increased self-esteem. | |

# Maurice, 36, lives in Alabama USA, Single, Jehovah's Witness

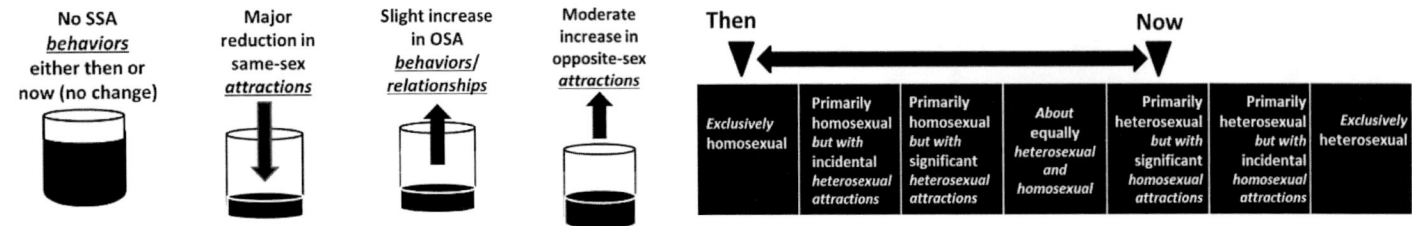

**SSA "then"**

I never really felt I was gay, even though I was attracted to the same sex. Those attractions were strong and overwhelming at times. I had no attractions to females. I never felt that it was sex I was after. I remember the excruciating pain I was in before discovering People Can Change. The pain was really intense, especially in my early 20s. I had nowhere to turn. I talked to members of my congregation and they had no advice. I was lost and even contemplated suicide. That was a really scary time for me. I was in an emotional tailspin.

**Motivations**

The gay community just didn't meet my needs. I didn't identify with gays. Sex between men just seemed like it was too much and was not what I was really looking for. I found the ex-gay community, and it seemed to better represent my identity as a man with same-sex attraction. These people help me feel whole and masculine. They help me to understand and successfully maintain healthy boundaries to meet my needs.

**SSA now**

I've learned how to meet my needs. I know what I want from other men. Probably the biggest change is in my view of women. Before, I felt I could and would never marry. I felt little if any attractions to the opposite sex. But now I feel confident that if I marry, I can have a good and successful marriage. This is a drastic change. It's even a drastic change in my identity. As a kid, I was confused. I did not understand my attractions or my feelings. Today, I feel like a regular man with some unmet emotional wounds. The clouds and fog have passed.

**What brought about change?**

Counseling did not help me. Religious experiences did nothing either. I just don't believe in faith healing. What helped me? The biggest benefit to me were *reading the books* and *doing the work*! To me, nothing beats self-understanding. I think it's better when I can read the books, accept what applies and reject what doesn't, and create my own path.

I heartily recommend Reparative Therapy of Male Homosexuality, by Nicolosi. Great book! Also, Battle for Normality. I *love* this book. It categorizes and gives extremely good names to feelings, emotions, and past experiences that I *never* thought I would be able to articulate. Without this book and its terminology, I would not be where I am! The other book is Coming Out Straight by Richard Cohen. It gave me the tools to put into practice all the stuff I had learned.

On top if that, People Can Change changed my life! None of this would be possible without the help of PCC. None of it!

It feels good to be a man among men, to feel accepted, to know that it's okay to be a male. It is so amazing to have same-sex attraction and *not feel ashamed!* I do not loathe or hate my same-sex attractions. I do not hate being "homosexual" as some would call me. I'm proud of who I am, and People Can Change has given that to me!

It has given me the ability—despite my religious community—to dignify myself and be proud of who I am! It has helped me find my identity! I now feel comfortable being a man. I have a community of people that is invaluable and with whom I can talk about these issues in a non-sexualized setting. I feel whole. The shame that I had is no more. I feel free!

| | |
|---|---|
| **Most helpful?** | Almost everything was beneficial. I have no complaints. |
| **Less helpful, or even harmful?** | Nothing was harmful. I've never felt pressured or pushed. Some admonishment was given from time to time but I did not feel unduly pressured in any way. I'm my own man and I can choose and not choose. I have exercised my choice numerous times. It was no big deal. |
| **Any other benefits?** | I have an identity, and one I can be proud of! I'm no longer confused, alone and wondering where my life is going. I'm proud to be a man. I'm proud of my same-sex attractions. I know some people don't feel that way, but I am. I'm a whole person. I have nothing to be ashamed of. |

I had always felt inferior and afraid of other men. I always thought I was different from them, and they couldn't and wouldn't understand. People Can Change helped me abolish those feelings! I am a man among men and equal to any man. I am competent and intelligent.

The benefits are so many, it's hard to keep count. It penetrates so much of my life. It affects how I deal with people, how I deal with a male boss, how I deal with people I look up to, how I deal with people I feel have it better than me, etc. I am *so much happier!* The fog and confusion are gone! I'm free!

# "Alex," 38, lives in Scotland, Heterosexually Married, Catholic

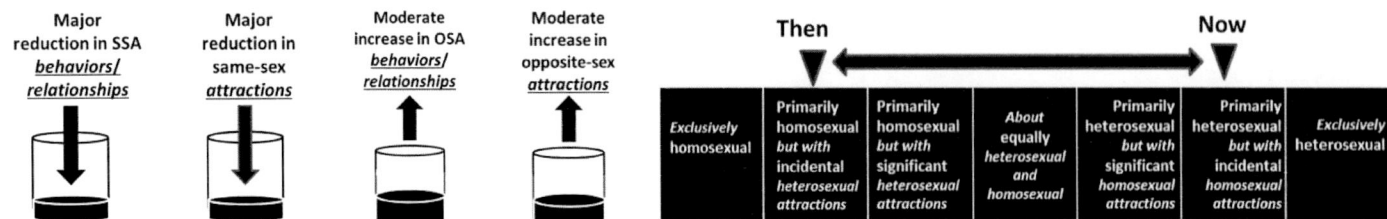

**SSA "then"**

I was never publicly "out." Most of my behavior was acting out to pornography and fantasy, with occasional interactions with other men. The addiction to pornography was what brought me to a 12 Step fellowship for people who had sex addiction. This was helpful, but did not address the issue completely. Many people in the fellowship advised me that I was probably just gay, and should embrace it. I felt they were not really listening to me. I believed at the time that I was heterosexual, but struggled with SSA frequently. I had girlfriends, and was able to have sex with a woman. But sometimes, I felt I wanted a man, and felt inferior to other men, whom I regarded as "real men."

**Motivations**

I have always known that this is not part of who I wanted to be. There was always something in me that was reluctant to go down the road of "coming-out," and for me it was more complicated than simply being gay. I am a man; I want to be a man; I like being a man. I knew that for me personally, same-sex attraction was a sexualized distortion of the person I wanted to be. Deficiencies in my own feelings of masculinity, along with a negative view of masculinity imposed on me from an early age, have made it difficult for me to identify with men and my inherent masculinity.

**SSA now**

I still have feelings of same-sex attraction but on a relatively infrequent basis. There has been a considerable reduction. Generally, when I experience SSA today, it is because there is something going wrong in my life, and I am reacting to this. I become absorbed in the attraction, but even the process of looking at what is happening is enough for those feelings to dissipate. Either I am feeling inadequate in my own masculinity, or I am frustrated by something. Occasionally I do look at pornography, but the frequency of this is considerably less than before. I have a good relationship with my girlfriend, who is aware of my difficulties in this area. When I feel secure in myself and my own masculinity, I experience an increase in attraction to the opposite sex. When I feel like a man, women become more beautiful, and I become more aware of their real femininity.

**What brought about change?**

Working the 12 Steps, reading literature on SSA, keeping in touch with other men, working a program and being honest with myself. Initially I had a few sessions with a counselor, who was of enormous help to me, particularly with working on my self-esteem, which I have continued since then. I made a point of becoming more involved in the world of men, while still being true to myself. I interact better with men, and feel more in tune with my own masculinity. I enjoy being a man today.

**Most helpful?**

Just being able to identify what I am going through has been enough to help me more than anything else. When I found People Can Change, I realized there were other people going through similar experiences, and there was a name for what I was going through! Even that knowledge was enough to make a huge difference in my life. In addition to that, I have found that the best thing for me has been to throw myself into being more involved with men (non-sexually, of course). If there is something I especially admire about a man, that's okay. It does not mean I am an inadequate man. So I can relate to other men far better than I used to.

**Less helpful, or even harmful?**

Telling people. Generally people do not understand, or are not really listening when I tell them, so I don't.

**Any other benefits?**

I have better self-esteem and am far more assertive. I am far less likely to be influenced by other people. Men I used to admire and fear I no longer see as demigods—they're just guys who have particular attributes I like. I can talk to them if I want and relate to them as equals.

I feel a greater sense of peace in my life, and even when things are not going well, I am normally able to identify the cause of discontentment, and accept what I cannot change.

I feel more at peace in my own body. I no longer consider myself less than other men, and even when I meet a man I previously would have feared and been attracted to, I can acknowledge his attributes, physical or otherwise, but not feel inferior to him.

I view women completely differently today. In some sense I find it harder to relate to them, as I don't understand them. But that's okay for me today. It's all right for me to not think like a woman. I don't have to be the good boy anymore, and I was not put on this earth to win their favor. There is nothing wrong with being a man and thinking and acting like one. I notice women now in a different way than I used to. I notice their femininity, and their differences—which can be both rewarding and infuriating at the same time!

# "Larry," 57, lives in Arizona. Heterosexually Married, Christian (Christian Science/eclectic)

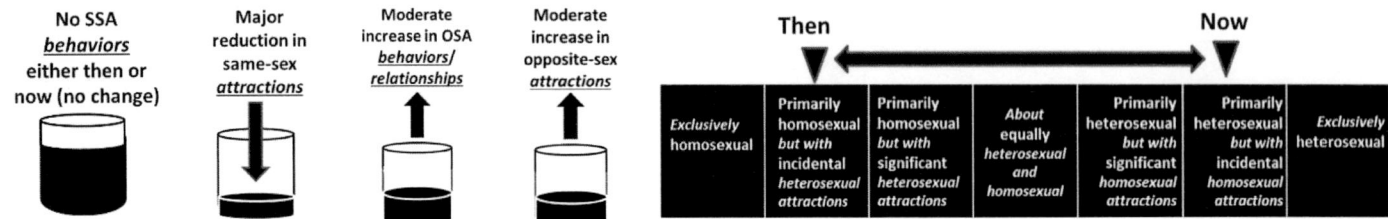

| | | | | | | |
|---|---|---|---|---|---|---|
| Exclusively homosexual | Primarily homosexual *but with incidental heterosexual attractions* | Primarily homosexual *but with significant heterosexual attractions* | *About equally* heterosexual *and* homosexual | Primarily heterosexual *but with significant homosexual attractions* | Primarily heterosexual *but with incidental homosexual attractions* | *Exclusively heterosexual* |

**SSA "then"**

It was troubling, because I felt jealous of other men and had low self-esteem. I felt I never had really joined the world of men. That has completely changed now. I never self-identified as gay, and never "acted out" with a man, and this, in my case, was protective.

**Motivations**

I had always compartmentalized my same-sex attractions. These attractions never felt like "me." In the wake of a relationship with a woman that ended badly a number of years ago, I felt my same-sex attractions move more front and center. I realized that I needed to decide if this was really "me" or if there was some other answer.

**SSA now**

Today, same-sex attractions are occasional and not nearly as compelling as they once were. If I experience them, they lift much more quickly than was once the case. I do experience opposite-sex attraction, yet it has a different, more holistic feel to it. I absolutely am sexually functional (and enjoy this immensely!) with my new wife. We married in the past two years, and we have a lovely, multi-dimensional relationship, of which sexual attraction is a part of the whole.

**What brought about change?**

I did a lot of personal work—reading books, etc., and finally discovered the Journey Into Manhood weekend, which is sponsored by People Can Change. That weekend was absolutely life-changing, and secured my journey toward a stronger identity of myself as a man. This in turn allowed for opposite-sex attractions to grow and same-sex attractions to diminish. I then had follow-up phone counseling with a man who was trained to help me continue my work in this area. I also participated in more advanced weekends offered by People Can Change, and became involved in the ManKind Project, completing its New Warrior Training Adventure and participating in an ongoing weekly men's group. Through all of this, I experienced a deeply rooted, organic shift away from same-sex attractions, and have claimed my identity as a man in a much stronger way. This to me has been a true gift!

**Most helpful?**

Without a doubt, the Journey Into Manhood weekend, and the follow-up phone coaching I pursued were the pivotal and most important activities. My ongoing association with thoughtful men in a men's group keeps me grounded in a good direction.

**Less helpful, or even harmful?**

My efforts to get clear on my sexual orientation (and there was definite work involved with this!) have been nothing but extremely positive—life-affirming, gender-affirming, and identity-affirming. I experienced absolutely NO negative effects from this. In contrast, staying on the path I was on would certainly have been very negative for me, personally.

**Any other benefits?**

My sense of myself as a man—who is just as salient as other men I admire—has been a huge shift. My self-esteem has soared, and my relationships with both men and women have improved greatly. I was married over a year ago to a beautiful, thoughtful woman. I am quite certain this would never have happened had it not been for my sexual-orientation changes.

**Final comment?**

Had I not felt free to pursue the avenues and organizations that have helped me in my journey to releasing same-sex attractions, I believe I may have become depressed and even suicidal.

# Charles, 25, lives in France and Turkey, Single, Spiritual "Believer" (But Non-Affiliated)

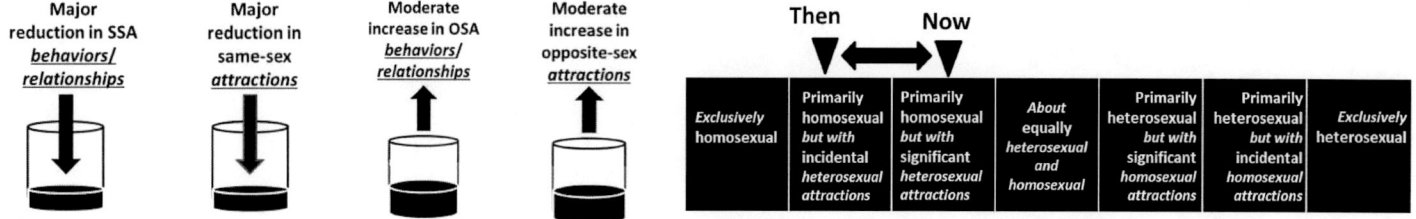

| Major reduction in SSA *behaviors/ relationships* | Major reduction in same-sex *attractions* | Moderate increase in OSA *behaviors/ relationships* | Moderate increase in opposite-sex *attractions* |

**SSA "then"**

When my first sexual attractions to men appeared as a teenager, I quickly realized what these phantasms were really about. It became obvious that this lust for older, strong and good-looking men matched the absence of and longing for my father who died when I was 2 years old. Living with a conflicted, frightening and burned-out mother—who was doing her best to raise four kids alone—I found in gay porn a "safe refuge" that brought me momentary comfort and excitement from a life I felt overwhelmed by. I had only a few anonymous sexual encounters, but I never felt pleased with and never identified with any "gay scene"—which seemed too far from what I really needed.

Being aware to some extent of the work I needed to do around men and in relationship to my mother, I started seeing a therapist at age 17. I saw three different psychotherapists for a few years, which helped me a lot in dealing with the relationship to my mother, peers, and family members—which were some of the issues underlying my SSA. However, the porn addiction and the attractions to men were still strong, and I felt regular psychotherapists were not trained to deal with such issues.

**Motivations**

I knowing that the loss of my father and the lack of brotherly connection when I was young will never be fulfilled by a sexual relationship to a man, and that precludes me from leading a gay life. I also strongly desire to find my soulmate of the opposite sex and to be a father.

**SSA now**

Two years after attending Journey into Manhood—although I still often feel drawn to men—I have realized this attraction is only seldom sexual, while being most of the time a longing for being closer to men I admire. SSA porn addiction has not vanished overnight but has sensibly diminished and has allowed me to actually feel sexual desire for the opposite sex in some situations. Although I have not yet been sexually involved with a woman, I surprise myself dreaming of being intimate with them, and see dating a woman as an exciting challenge.

**What brought about change?**

At age 23, I decided to attend Journey Into Manhood in England – which I had learned about on the Internet. This 48-hour workshop was a breakthrough like no other I had experienced in years of "regular therapy." The challenging environment of experienced men and the sense of brotherhood provided me with a safe place to do work. Releasing all the shame around these unwanted attractions that I had never told anyone about, and being accepted just I am, was a life-changing experience. The community of committed men with whom I have kept in touch ever since is a great source of mutual support and reaching out when feeling down.

I view this journey as a life-long journey, and have kept working on issues underlying SSA or its symptoms. Staffing a JiM retreat, working around the feminine by attending the Noble Man weekend by Celebration of Being, taking part in weekly group counseling, establishing mutual support-based accountability relationships with peers who experiencing the same issue—all have helped me tremendously in feeling a whole man among men.

**Most helpful?**

Attending workshops such as JiM or Noble Man have been life-changing experiences. Regular support groups and strong authentic friendships are also needed, as this journey is not one that is done alone, but continuously supported by others.

| | |
|---|---|
| **Less helpful, or even harmful?** | I have found the "religious/conservative vs liberal/progressive" politically oriented divide misleading and detrimental to anyone experiencing same-sex attraction—be it self-identified gays or SSA men seeking change. Any politician, religious leader, and pseudo non-profit organization that claims to hold the truth—but that really knows nothing about SSA-struggling men—has no right or legitimacy to take hostage the debate for its own purposes. On the other hand, any organization that seeks to prevent same-sex-attracted men from experiencing depression over those attractions or even from committing suicide should be left in peace, or else supported—regardless of which path men ultimately choose (living a gay life or seeking change). |
| **Any other benefits?** | Healing my wounds towards my mother and my brother, being in an authentic, assertive yet loving relationship to them, making deeper friendship are some of the important processes that are going on since I have started therapy. |
| | The wonderful transformations I have been witnessing around me and all the loving compassion and support I have seen in the community of men seeking change have increased my spirituality. |

# "Joe," 53, lives in Ohio USA, Divorced, Catholic

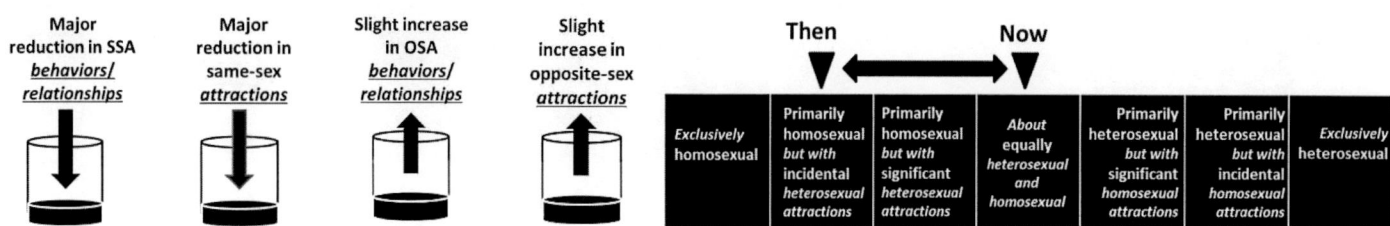

| SSA "then" | While I was married, I had numerous anonymous encounters with men. It was an all-consuming part of my life. When I look back at that time in my life, I now realize just how much time, effort, and money I expended for instant gratification. I was religious in name only, not authentically connected to God. I was a horrible example for my family, and unfortunately, I went through a divorce because of my actions |
| --- | --- |
| **Motivations** | First and foremost, homosexuality is against my personal religious beliefs. Second, I wanted to improve my connection with my children and family. And lastly, I wanted to feel better about myself. |
| **SSA now** | My SSA is a part of me, and it will always be a part of me. Now, the difference is that I can control it and keep it in its proper place in my life rather than letting it run everything. I have substituted other positive things in place of constantly dwelling on my SSA. |
| **What brought about change?** | Professional therapy, pastoral counseling, religious ministries, <u>People Can Change</u>, experiential personal-growth programs. |
| **Most helpful?** | The <u>Journey Into Manhood</u> weekend was the most dramatic effort I took. Spending a weekend being challenged by other men who cared was instrumental in my journey. |
| **Less helpful, or even harmful?** | Spending time at an Exodus conference where there was a "pray away the gay" attitude was not very helpful. |
| | I have never felt forced to seek <u>reparative therapy</u>. This is something that I have done on my own. I have the right to seek help any way I feel is right. Just because I have SSA does not mean that I have to live a gay lifestyle. I have choices. They are my choices; others have the right to choose other courses of action. |
| **Any other benefits?** | Because of my efforts, I am a more confident man; one who is not so judgmental of others. I have more of a quiet self-confidence that others have noticed. I have become a much better father to my children because I am more understanding and patient. |

# Samuel, 38, lives in South Africa, Single, Christian (Pentecostal)

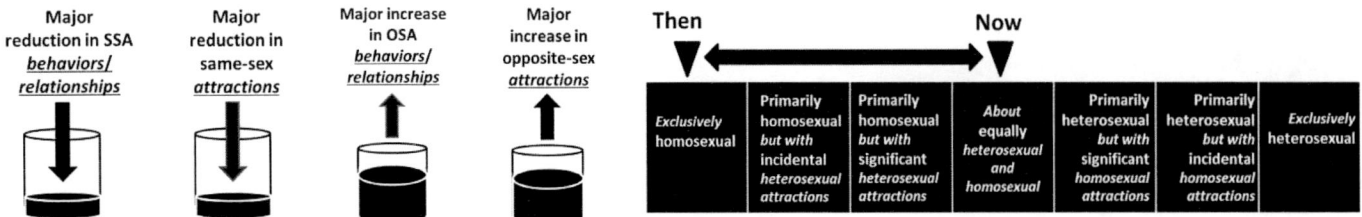

| | | | | Then | | | | Now | | | |
|---|---|---|---|---|---|---|---|---|---|---|---|

**SSA "then"**

From the age of 19, I lived an active homosexual life. I was in same-sex relationships. I was addicted to cocaine and drank a lot. I believe this was because I knew that I was living a life of sin. I grew up in a Christian home with strong moral standards but fell into a life of homosexuality. I believe this was because I always felt I was not like other guys. Also, when I was younger, I was abused by an older boy.

I was in this lifestyle until the age of 29, when I was in an abusive relationship with a man. I realized God did not want me to live this way and that He has more for me.

**Motivations**

My belief in God and my personal convictions. I knew that I was living a lie and that the only way out was to seek God and then to participate in counseling.

**SSA now**

I still have some attraction to the same sex, but also some attraction to the opposite sex. I have not been sexually active for the past seven years. I still have SSA feelings now and again, but it is like any other kind of recovery—after you are out of it you still get urges but you choose not to act on them.

**What brought about change?**

I had counseling and a support system around me, mostly with strong males in my life. I also got involved in counseling others and helping with a street ministry and working with prostitutes and helping them. Helping others helped me. All the help I received, I did so through the church that I am part of.

**Most helpful?**

The fact that those around me did not judge me but they just wanted to help me.

**Less helpful, or even harmful?**

My work was in night clubs, so I had to resign my position and go into another business. Also unhelpful: some old friendships that I had to break off.

**Any other benefits?**

I was suicidal when I was in that lifestyle, but after I got out of it I have found that I am happier and more relaxed in my life.

I believe that I have grown as a man and that I have become more masculine. I have also seen that my friendships with other men are real friendships, and that I do not feel any sexual connection with them.

# Charles, 40, lives in Ohio USA, Heterosexually Married, Christian (Anglican)

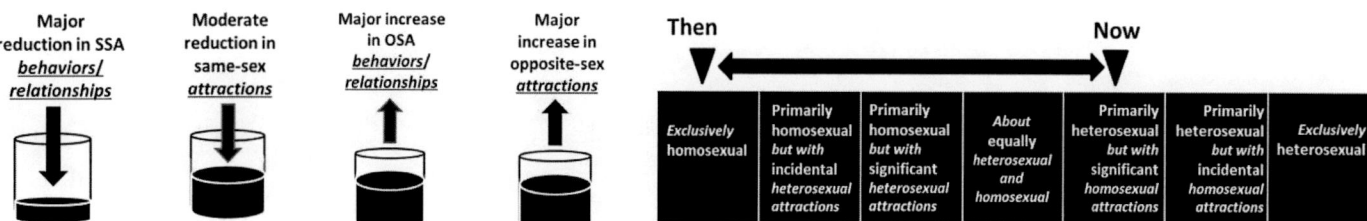

**SSA "then"**

Before beginning my journey, I experienced intense feelings of SSA. I lived a fairly closeted life, a double life as a Christian who was "acting out" in secret. I had next to no opposite-sex attraction, and I was miserably conflicted. I desired intimate connection with men, but I also desired marriage to a woman. I became desperate for change when I began secretly "acting out" with men after having been married for four years.

**Motivations**

Though same-sex attraction was never a choice, I have always felt that it was in conflict with the person that I truly am. I am a Christian who believes that homosexuality is not God's best for mankind. I am a husband and father of four now, and if I had believed the lie that homosexuality was my only option or that I was born that way, I would not have pursued marriage and fatherhood, which have been the two most wonderful experiences of my life. Since being married, I still struggle with unwanted same-sex attractions, but remaining a husband and father is a strong motivation for me to continue my journey away from SSA.

**SSA now**

I am not sexually active with men at all. I am extremely attracted to my wife and desire her sexually. I still experience SSA, but the intensity is far less than in the past, and I can more easily put these attractions in perspective, realizing that I need healthy non-sexual connection with men—which, when that need doesn't get met, shows up for me as SSA or body envy.

When I have participated in experiential men's weekends, such as Journey Into Manhood, as well as in the days or weeks following, I have temporarily experienced a COMPLETE elimination of SSA. While these feelings, attractions and desires have later resurfaced, their power is much less, and I then realize that I have not been actively engaging in my journey and need to re-calibrate.

**What brought about change?**

I have been in counseling in which my counselor used a variety of counseling approaches including reparative therapy. I have also attended two experiential weekends, Journey Into Manhood and Edge Venture, and I have staffed such weekends, as well. I also have been a part of support groups such as Exodus International,[10] Homosexuals Anonymous and Celebrate Recovery.

**Most helpful?**

By far, the most helpful and healing have been my involvement with men's experiential weekends, like Edge Venture and Journey Into Manhood. But also, having a professional counselor who supported my desire for change and communicated hope every step of the way.

**Less helpful, or even harmful?**

Less helpful for me was my involvement in 12 Step support groups. This form of support just doesn't resonate for me like experiential and psychodynamic work.

**Any other benefits?**

I have learned to assert myself and to not allow myself to be taken advantage of. I have improved as a husband and father, with incredible confidence. I have learned to relate to other men as a man among men, rather than seeing myself as less-than or unworthy of masculine love and affirmation. I feel like a man, and for the first time in my life, I am actually thankful to be a man.

---

[10] Succeeded by Restored Hope Network (http://restoredhopenetwork.org/)

# Kevin, 40, lives in California USA, Single, Christian

| Major reduction in SSA *behaviors/ relationships* | Moderate reduction in same-sex *attractions* | Slight increase in OSA *behaviors/ relationships* | Moderate increase in opposite-sex *attractions* | Then ⟷ Now | | | | | | |
|---|---|---|---|---|---|---|---|---|---|---|
| ⬇ | ⬇ | ⬆ | ⬆ | ▼ ⟷ ▼ | | | | | | |
| | | | | *Exclusively* homosexual | Primarily homosexual *but with incidental heterosexual attractions* | Primarily homosexual *but with significant heterosexual attractions* | *About equally heterosexual and homosexual* | Primarily heterosexual *but with significant homosexual attractions* | Primarily heterosexual *but with incidental homosexual attractions* | *Exclusively heterosexual* |

**SSA "then"**
I started being voluntarily sexually active around 11 to 12 years old and was sexually active in my teenage years through adulthood. It was most difficult to deal with in my late 20s to early 30s, and that's when I felt like I went off the "deep end" emotionally. At my worst, I was hooking up with men as often as four to five times a week—usually different men.

**Motivations**
I have taken steps to reduce my same-sex-attraction because my goal is to be a Biblical Christian. I knew that underneath my SSA were wounds that I didn't know what to do with. I was sexually abused as a pre-teen (9 to 11 years old) by an uncle, and I could sense that my desire for men increased dramatically, mainly because my need for attention and acceptance escalated.

**SSA now**
Since my experiences with Journey Into Manhood, I went from being extremely promiscuous to no sexual activity with men. My attractions are completely manageable at this point. I am still dominantly attracted to men, but my attraction to women has gone up from zero to actually believing and feeling that I can get married; very exciting, yet scary proposition.

**What brought about change?**
I have received years of in-church counseling, but the MOST effective venture I've ever undertaken is Journey Into Manhood! My life completely changed after attending. It was the first time I didn't feel "tortured" about who I am, first time that I felt shame-free, and the first time I felt authentic. I experienced intense healing and I no longer "bottle" or hide my SSA, but rather I'm super open about it with friends. They have been ultra-supportive, and my connection with them has deepened.

Theoretically, even if I were to decide one day to enter into a same-sex relationship, it would not be for the same reasons I had before I experienced Journey Into Manhood. Those were based on unmet core needs, unresolved wounds, and so on. Today I feel free to fall in love for the right reasons—unconditional love for another human being.

Since attending Journey Into Manhood, I noticed that my heart now seeks a woman more when it comes to finding a life partner, and rarely a man. Yes, when I'm triggered, I'm tempted to connect with men in a sexual way, but those are not meaningful interactions for me; they are more like medication for pain. I don't want to sound judgmental by the way: I do believe gay men can fall in love and be completely invested. It's simply not the direction my heart is telling me to go.

**Most helpful?**
Journey Into Manhood helped me heal, become more authentic and resolve intense amounts of shame. I have never experienced such freedom and acceptance.

**Less helpful, or even harmful?**
NONE!

**Any other benefits?**
Yes, I have been able to help others in my church with SSA. The counseling is not really about the SSA but more about a healthy connection to masculinity, meeting needs in authentic ways versus inauthentic ways (e.g., gay porn), connecting with God as a God of grace and not of judgment, etc.

# Stefan, 41, lives in Germany, Single, Catholic

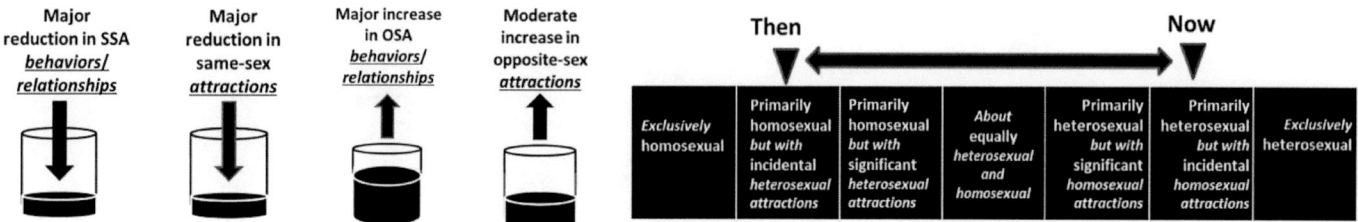

| | |
|---|---|
| **SSA "then"** | Between 14 and 35, I was sexually addicted to pornography, sex with many different men, and masturbation. I became totally concentrated on the idealized body of the other man. Being allowed to be close to him always meant to do anything he desired. I lived this secretly, had a coming out only with close friends. I was been unhappy with all this: my sexuality, my shame about my own body and manhood, my compulsive desire for the body of other men. |
| **Motivations** | I realized that my homosexual desires were an escape from my self-hatred and shame, from real friendships with other men and their emotions, and from women. I realized that I used sex only to reduce distress and not because of real love and relationship. I wanted to live as the man God had created me to be, at peace with his desires, and at peace with other men and women. |
| **SSA now** | I now fall in love with and desire women! Sometimes I still idealize bodies of other men, but I am able then to understand my wounded self and no longer need to compensate with sexuality. I have sex with women and feel much safer in their presence today. |
| **What brought about change?** | Counseling, psychotherapy, and experiential trainings like Journey Into Manhood or other trainings concentrating on the development of my male identity. I learned to understand my emotions, deal with my emotions, show and share emotions. I learned to be authentic in relationships with men and women. I worked through traumatic experiences and distress. I learned to accept my own body and my own manhood. I learned to accept others, love others and to overcome fear. |
| **Most helpful?** | I needed the mixture of all the support—groups, therapist, counselor, trainings. |
| **Less helpful, or even harmful?** | Nothing. |
| **Any other benefits?** | Self-esteem, authentic relationships, emotions, inner sense of masculinity. |

# David, 41, lives in Arizona USA, Single, Agnostic.

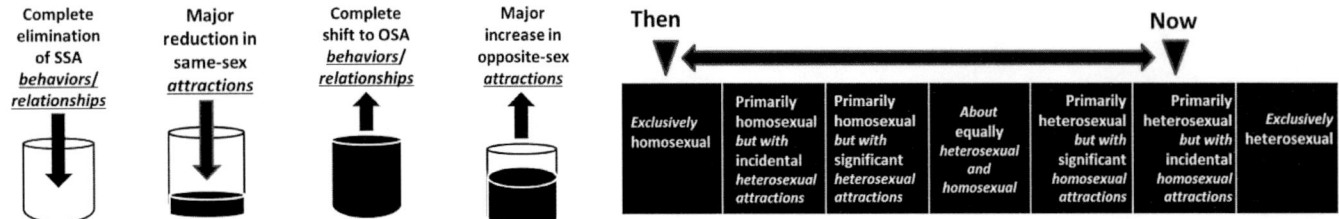

| | | |
|---|---|---|
| **SSA "then"** | In my teens, I was exclusively attracted to men. In my 20s, I was married to another man. In my 30s, I decided to re-identify as heterosexual and began to date women. Today, I date women exclusively. |
| **Motivations** | I desired a life that was more compatible with my personal goals as far as family, marriage, children, etc. |
| **SSA now** | I have had no interest in dating other men since 2003. Currently, I am very happy and functional in a heterosexual relationship. Romantic feelings toward my girlfriend were present immediately when we met, and the sexual desires I have toward her are equal to those I once had for men when I was pursuing a homosexual lifestyle. With her, I feel genuinely and completely fulfilled emotionally, spiritually, and sexually.<br><br>Now, all of my sexual fantasies and desires are heterosexual in nature. My SSA is only strong enough to notice an attractive man. I do not sexually fantasize about men, nor do I pursue them romantically. I am moderately sexually active today, but only heterosexually. All of my sexual fantasies and desires are heterosexual in nature. |
| **What brought about change?** | Changes in attitudes and behaviors. This was done completely on my own. I have never attended any counseling, retreats, or 12 Step programs. |
| **Any other benefits?** | I feel a heightened self-esteem due to my sense of accomplishment. Also, as a functioning heterosexual, I feel a stronger sense of manhood, which I lacked previously. |
| **Final comment?** | A gay life works great for some people. I don't see any negative effects of taking a gay-affirming path if that's what a person feels is best for him. In my case, it did not work for me and it was not the best approach for me to take. For that reason, I made the effort to become heterosexual.<br><br>Certainly, sexual-orientation change is possible and for some people does happen. I think that what adults choose to do with their lives should be their own business. That includes joining support groups consisting of others with the same goals. |

# "Richard," 45, lives in Oregon USA, Heterosexually Married, Christian

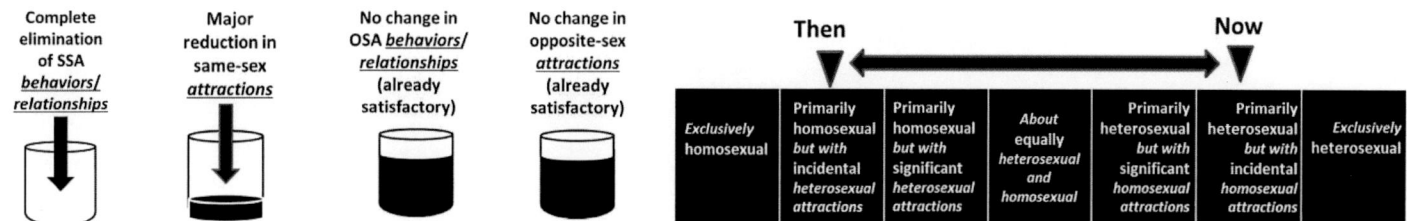

**SSA "then"**

I was deeply closeted, since I was married and a worship leader at our church. But I wouldn't go a day without fantasies about men and sex with men filling my mind. I felt drawn to pornography and would spend excessive time masturbating. This affected my marriage as well as my productivity at work. I also would seek out anonymous men for sexual encounters at least weekly for over 10 years. I was extremely unhappy and conflicted, but I felt no choice about these attractions and thought there was no way for me to deal with them in a healthy way. I couldn't turn them off and I couldn't live without them. It was a living hell. I knew I needed to find a way to get help and to become real. I didn't know at that time if that would mean leaving my wife and embracing the gay lifestyle or finding a way to deal with my attractions and compulsions.

**Motivations**

I had been aware of same-sex attractions before puberty, so it was my baseline sexual identity, but it never felt right for me. At the same time that I was sexually attracted to men, I was deeply emotionally attracted and connected to women, which is what drove my dating and marriage to my best friend. This did not stop my SSA however, and I knew I needed to better understand my attractions to understand myself. I entered into this process of my own free will and out of the desire to know myself more fully and to be able to finally live as a whole-hearted, authentic man, with no need or desire to hide any parts of my life, thoughts or feelings anymore.

**SSA now**

I only occasionally have a flicker of same-sex sexual attraction now. I never have sexual attraction for men I know, because I've found that a real-life connection is so much deeper and more fulfilling. I have not had sexual encounters with other men for over nine years and have not used pornography in over five. My sexual relationship with my wife is mutually enjoyable and feels more natural than ever. I do not find myself being sexually attracted to other women, but I do more deeply appreciate the ways in which they are different from me. I used to feel much more in common with women than with other men, though I never thought of myself as a woman. Now I feel fully masculine and realize that masculinity is a spectrum, not simply the hyper-masculinized stereotypes portrayed in the media.

The sight of a physically attractive man used to immediately trigger sexual arousal and fantasies. Now I see another man, much like myself, with physical characteristics that I either identify with or admire. I also see a whole person, with a history, with relationships, with faults, not just a physical image. I have learned that I need intimate, healthy, emotionally connected relationships with other men. As I have taken the steps to be open and vulnerable with the men in my life, I am growing in these relationships. This is filling the void in my heart that I used to medicate with gay porn or acting out sexually with other men. The real connection I long for with other men is not sexual or romantic, but pure, brotherly affection, affirmation and belonging.

**What brought about change?**

I found a trusted group of friends who embraced both me and my wife when I shared my story with them, and my journey began to move toward internal healing for my heart and healing for our marriage. My recovery initially focused on the sexual compulsions and addictions related to porn and "acting out," and it moved into the arena of SSA and healing my wounded masculinity over the next three to four years.

I have attended two separate experiential weekend intensives by two different organizations, one specifically to deal with unwanted SSA and the other more focused on wholeness in masculinity from a Christian perspective. Both helped immeasurably in opening my eyes and heart to how fully masculine I am and in allowing me to connect with my authentic emotions, needs and desires. The follow-up work I have done has included online support groups, individual counseling, my own study and journaling, as well as purposeful entering into the community of men through local men's groups.

**Most helpful?**

The experiential weekends sponsored by People Can Change (Journey Into Manhood) and The Samson Society (48 Hours Intensive) were completely transformational for me. Their effect on my inner and outer life was exclusively positive. I came away with a deeper sense of who I was and how I fit into the world of men, as well as how I could better relate to the women in my life. They were the first time I experienced healthy deep connection with other men and also the first time I was able to access deeply locked emotions without raging or damaging myself or others.

Individual counseling has helped me slowly peel back the layers of lies I've told myself, and to take steps to proactively live my own life with purpose. That has opened up the possibility of living life as a part of the community of men through my own engagement and even leadership in men's groups. They have become my lifeblood as far as building and maintaining healthy male friendships and connection.

**Less helpful, or even harmful?**

No. I often had thoughts of suicide and depression before seeking to understand and change my attractions. I have NEVER had a suicidal thought since beginning that process. This journey to greater awareness and authenticity has been like stepping from a dark grave into the light of day and fresh air!

I have experienced no harmful effects from any interventions I have tried. The only harm in my life related to same-sex attractions was the years I spent denying, repressing and "acting out" in dangerous ways on those attractions.

**Any other benefits?**

I feel so much more authentic. My relationships have grown in depth since my change efforts. I have learned to stop identifying myself by my attractions, but by my worth as a man. I feel completely comfortable with other men, even men who do not share my interests or abilities. I know that I am fully a man, regardless of my attributes. I have had greater confidence, which has expanded my horizons professionally as I have been able to step up in leadership as I felt led and also to express myself assertively in situations that I felt needed to change. I feel like a whole person, a whole man for the first time in my life.

**Final comments?**

Anyone should be able to seek *of their own free will* a course of action that does not harm another person. In my experience, efforts to change my sexual attractions have been overwhelmingly positive. If it is not unethical to support a transgendered person's choice to change their physical gender to match their internal experience, how can it be unethical to support a person who desires to change their internal experience to more closely match their morals, ethics or beliefs?

# "Nathan," 32, lives in Maryland USA, Single, Jewish

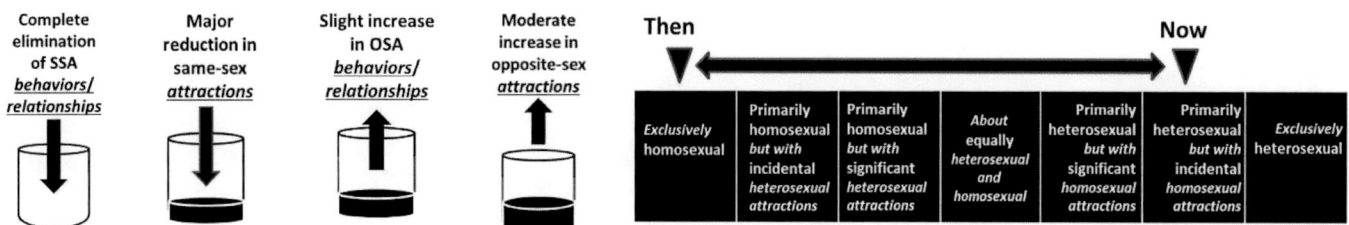

**SSA "then"**

I was closeted and never told a soul about this. The shame was huge. I ignored the issue for many years, and "acted out" sexually during my teenage years, but always in secret—which only made the shame even stronger. I am stubborn, and there was no way that I would ever consider "coming out." Every time I read that that was my only option, I became depressed.

**Motivations**

I have always wanted to form a family with a wife and kids. I grew up with a grandmother and a grandfather, a mother, a father (although he wasn't around), and an uncle and an aunt. This was what always seemed normal and that's what I wanted for myself and continue to want. No one suggested to me I should receive therapy, but rather, when I became desperate, I did my own research to pursue the only therapy that gave me some level of hope. At that point, I was addicted to gay porn, and I had already hooked up with a stranger. I hit a low and wanted change in my life. My family has no religious beliefs, and my mom would support me if I decided to be openly gay. Even my friends would embrace me.

**SSA now**

I don't feel same-sex attractions in my everyday life as I used to. At times I notice an attractive guy and think he is good looking, but this is no longer sexual. I go to the gym every day and see naked guys with muscular and athletic bodies and do not feel at all sexually attracted.

I am no longer involved in sexual addictions. The only porn that I want now is straight porn (girls). Whereas before this therapy, I tried all sorts of filters to control my porn addiction (with little success), today I feel fully empowered to decide for myself what activities to get involved with. Even with no filters, I have zero temptation to watch gay porn. I see it as boring and I am not tempted.

I would say that I have experienced a radical elimination of SSA. I do not notice guys around me, I do not feel interested in gay porn, and I prefer connecting to guys as friends. I suppose I could still enjoy sexual intimacy with guys, but I am at peace with that; my goals in this therapy were never to be totally un-attracted to guys. But today I am more likely to notice a girl out there than a guy.

**What brought about change?**

I read a book about this therapy called <u>Coming Out Straight</u>. It directly depicted my life (no father present, too close to mom). The book made total sense to me. That led me to start psychotherapy, and that changed my life.

**Less helpful, or even harmful?**

Nothing was harmful. It might have been hard work but not harmful. Not having this option would have been harmful.

**Any other benefits?**

I am definitely more confident. I am less of a victim. I am more in touch with my emotions. I am no longer ashamed of my sexuality—and for the first time started being authentic about it to friends and family. I was able to come out in my own terms to those who I wanted to tell. I am better able to connect with men. I am a more loving person. And I have become less judgmental, even to the extent of supporting the freedom of gay marriage, while not wanting that for myself.

# Robert, 47, lives in Texas USA, Heterosexually Married, Christian

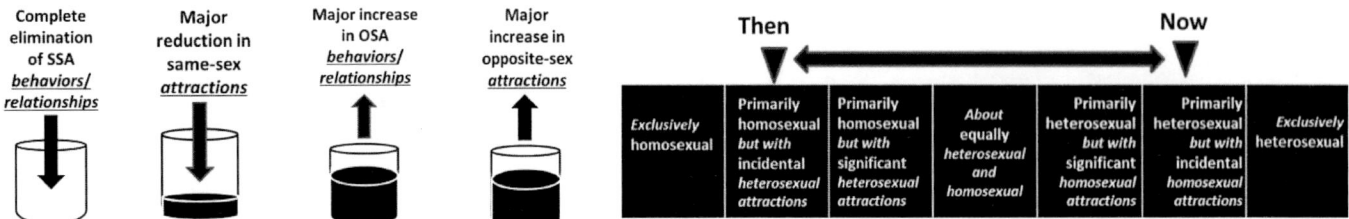

**SSA "then"**

In my early 20s, I was having sexual relations with men on a regular basis. I did not feel it was the right choice for me, but I did not know how to channel my sexual feelings toward women. At this time, I spent most of my time with a group of friends who lived a gay lifestyle. I never came out publicly, but I did my best to embrace the lifestyle that went with the behavior of having sex with men. I was very conflicted, and came to the point of being suicidal. I was very unhappy and started using drugs and alcohol to try to feel better. This made it worse.

**Motivations**

My belief that God does not want me to live in a homosexual lifestyle. Because of this, I never felt 100% at home during the time I lived that lifestyle. It never seemed to fit with who I am made to be, but I had addictive drives to continue the behaviors, even though they made me feel guilty and shameful. Since beginning the journey out of sexualized same-sex attraction, I have found more peace and satisfaction than I ever thought possible.

**SSA now**

Most of the time, I don't have sexual feelings for men. Occasionally, when I feel insecure or emotionally hurt, I may find myself having sexual feelings toward men. I have learned to go back to the root cause and address it. This works for me. I am now happily married and feel very sexually attracted to her. My SSA today happens occasionally, when I am triggered emotionally by events at work that make me feel insecure about myself as a man. It has been eight years since I had sex with men on a regular basis, and it has now been over two years since my last encounter with a man.

**What brought about change?**

Counseling (approximately five years), church sponsored ministries, a support group for men struggling with unwanted SSA, experiential weekends designed to help with understanding and changing the drives toward same-sex attractions.

**Most helpful?**

The experiential weekends sponsored by <u>People Can Change</u>.

**Less helpful, or even harmful?**

Well-meaning friends and family who told me to "just stop."

**Any other benefits?**

The biggest secondary benefit would be my education. Before beginning the journey, I had tried to go to college, but due to my emotional turmoil had not been able to finish. After beginning the journey, I came to a place of emotional healing significant enough to allow me to complete a bachelor's degree, and am currently in my third year of graduate school. Also, the more I feel in touch with my own masculinity, the better I am able to relate to my wife, and that has greatly improved our marriage.

**Final comment?**

I was so conflicted before my change efforts, that I became seriously suicidal. Attempting to live and embrace a homosexual lifestyle was very damaging to me. Since learning that change is possible, and beginning my own personal journey, I have experienced increasing peace of mind, improved self-esteem, and no suicidal thoughts.

# "Hakim," 24, lives in United Arab Emirates, Single, Muslim

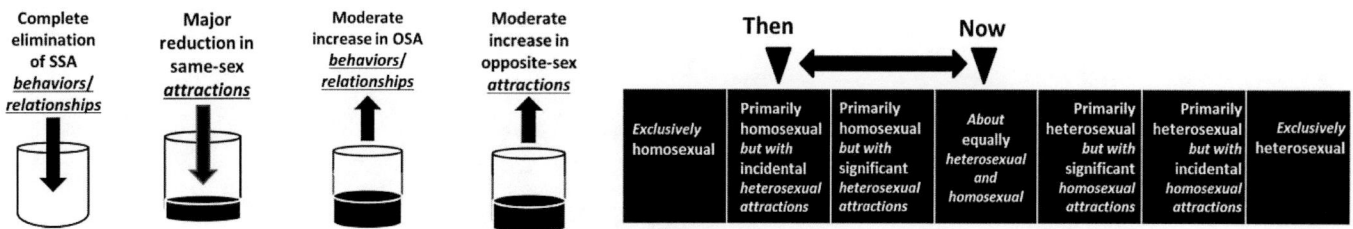

**SSA "then"**

After high school, when I was living in Sweden, I decided I would come out to everyone as gay—and I did, quite literally. I came out on national television because I had been approached by a documentary producer who was interested in my story. In those days I was particularly conflicted because apart from my own aversion to SSA, my parents were religious Muslims. Eventually I self-identified as gay, thus giving free reign to what was at first unwanted SSA and in a sense still was unwanted but I had stopped resisting. At university, I started engaging in gay sex. My life went from bad to worse. Starting off with mild depression and anxiety before self-identification, I was a 19-year-old living the so-called gay lifestyle but suffering from severe anxiety attacks. I lost interest in everything. I felt I had sacrificed myself for an addiction.

**Motivations**

My life was rapidly deteriorating. My mental health was suffering. I was depressed, anxious and had panic attacks. I had lost contact with my family. I was riddled with inner conflicts and was extremely unhappy as a result. I knew that I was living an unhealthy lifestyle that I had to change.

**SSA now**

I used to think SSA was the problem, but I now know that I have underlying issues and SSA is just a symptom of these core issues. Before, it was something that was overwhelming, whereas now it is something that I'm in control of. It still exists but to a considerably lesser degree. These days, SSA is more like my barometer of psychological well-being. When I experience increased SSA it alerts me to a problem area in my life that I need to address. When I deal with that lack, the SSA again subsides. The strength of my SSA indicates to me how much of a man I feel I am, at a given moment. When I make the choices that are conducive to my psychological well-being, then I can go without experiencing any SSA whatsoever. Instead I experience identification with other men, and consequently experience increased opposite-sex attraction. When I'm not doing what I need to do for self-care, again I notice the appearance of SSA.

**What brought about change?**

As I had no access to expert therapists, I had to rely on their books. I owe most of my progress (out of SSA) to "Bibliotherapy," or books by various psychologists. I have followed the advice given and have experienced remarkable change in the positive direction. I am more confident in myself because I have learned about my weaknesses, and I'm taking steps to address them. As a result I can identify with other men and be more confident with the opposite sex.

**Most helpful?**

Good to be able to talk to other people in the same situation with whom I can exchange advice.

**Less helpful, or even harmful?**

Nothing was harmful.

**Any other benefits?**

Nothing turned out to be directly related to sexual attractions. My focus has primarily been on how to overcome my sense of inferiority and lack of identification with other men, which reflects on the surface as SSA. My self-confidence and identification with other men, my physical health, my mental health, my empathy and the quality of my interpersonal relationships have all improved immensely.

# Jose, 26, lives in Mexico, Single, Catholic

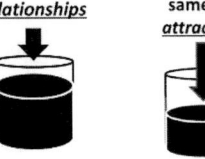 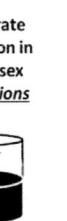 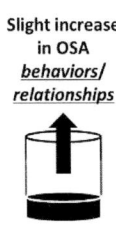 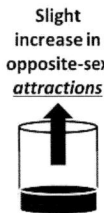 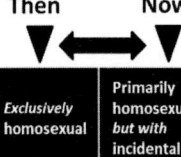

| Slight reduction in SSA *behaviors/ relationships* | Moderate reduction in same-sex *attractions* | Slight increase in OSA *behaviors/ relationships* | Slight increase in opposite-sex *attractions* |
|---|---|---|---|

| Then | | Now | | | | |
|---|---|---|---|---|---|---|
| *Exclusively homosexual* | *Primarily homosexual but with incidental heterosexual attractions* | *Primarily homosexual but with significant heterosexual attractions* | *About equally heterosexual and homosexual* | *Primarily heterosexual but with significant homosexual attractions* | *Primarily heterosexual but with incidental homosexual attractions* | *Exclusively heterosexual* |

**SSA "then"**

I discovered I had SSA when I was 14. I felt awful because I did not understand why. From that age until I was 22, I lived believing that someday this would disappear, that time would erase it. During those eight years I lived a life of despair, feeling misunderstood and unhappy. I saw only two options: living a gay life, which would take me away from my values, beliefs, family, etc., or suppressing my feelings. Oh, what a lie! I later learned I don't need to suppress but fulfill those needs in a healthy, non-sexual way.

**Motivations**

I want to change because I want to find the joy that I have not glimpsed in the gay environment. I firmly believe that what I want and really need is to fulfill my needs in healthy non-sexual ways. Also my values, my beliefs and God are very important reasons to seek change. However, they would be of no importance if they were not taking me to an immense joy and true inner peace that I have experienced whenever I'm authentic with myself and follow what I believe is the truth and above all what my heart invites me to seek: change, healing and true love.

**SSA now**

Three years ago, I searched on the Internet "I don't want to be gay" and first came across the truth—something that made sense in my life: root causes and A MANS Journey in the website of People Can Change. Since I started therapy, I began a path to greater peace and happiness.

Therapy and healing weekends have not only helped me to see my problems differently but to see myself as someone who is good and valuable and acceptable just as I am—even unchanged.

**What brought about change?**

I have learned from my own experience that I can overcome homosexual desires by creating a support network, having men around me who can help me heal underlying emotional pain and who support me and help me feel true love. The hardest thing in my journey has been finding this support network, mainly because of the misinformation there is in our society about SSA. In the last months, I began to form a support network which I believe has been essential to help me find peace and joy instead of looking for them in same-sex relations where I never found them.

**Most helpful?**

Seeing that other men have already changed and that they are authentic and happy.

**Less helpful, or even harmful?**

I went to a therapist who did not believe in change and did not respect my decision to change. He wanted me to live a gay life. After four sessions, I left him.

**Any other benefits?**

I have gained self-esteem, confidence, peace, clarity, and have improved my relations with friends; I've learned how to relate to other men and women in a healthier way, feeling part of a world of men, feeling the same as them.

# Dan, 49, lives in South Carolina USA, Widowed, Christian

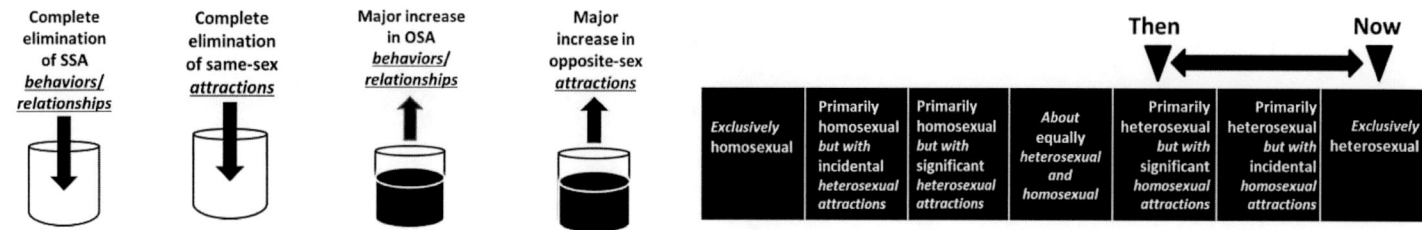

**SSA "then"**

I was miserable. I was raped by a man when I was a high school student, when my first encounter looking for adult love went terribly wrong. My early 20s brought a potentially lethal cancer into my life and a year of chemo. After surviving cancer, I met my wife to be.

We fell in love and were married for nearly nine years, and had two children. Although I loved my wife, the need and longing to be understood, loved, and valued by another man could only be fulfilled by the friendship of another man. I had grown up ignorant and starving in all things healthy with men. After my wife died, I felt like I had to let myself explore a gay life. I moved in with a male partner, even though I knew the day that I moved in, that I would eventually move out. I felt trapped. I cared about "Bob," but I believed I had to give it a try, or I would never know.

Although I cared for him, in all honesty the relationship was just about sex because the sex brought us closer, and because it was really the touch and physical closeness that I wanted. When Bob refused counseling, that was my way out to return to my Christian faith and a God that I knew loved me and was committed to me as his wounded child.

However, that recovery would be a rocky road. I dove into a deeper drug lifestyle to escape feeling my negative feelings. That, and the isolation and the inability to connect, nearly took my life, until a friend from Nate Larkin's Samson Society recommended Journey Into Manhood, and that, along with my counselor John, began the impetus for me to self-direct my own pursuit of happiness. I begin to reclaim my masculinity and seek the life and healing that I desired, and deserved to seek. I was well on my way to having my life back.

**Motivations**

Initially, my motivations were spiritual in nature. I accepted that the roots of my unwanted SSA were not a spiritual issue, but that of a wounded boy who had never had a healthy, nurturing fathering, and were profoundly emotional and psychological in nature. My marriage, depression, my religious convictions and recognizing my own right to personal happiness are what motivated me to pursue change. After my second suicide attempt, I knew I had to get help. Family Strategies & Coaching (Arizona) and People Can Change changed my life and gave me strategies to live the life I always wanted to live.

**SSA now**

Today I am able to recognize beauty in both the masculine and feminine. Initially, being aware of same-sex attraction was very troubling to me. However, it is then that I am reminded that I have intrinsic healthy needs that are a part of a man's life, and will be for the rest of my life, just as with any other man, regardless.

**What brought about change?**

When I quit using meth and stopped abusing alcohol, I was able to see things more clearly. I wanted to like and love myself as a man of value for my good. I began to like myself again, and I didn't need the approval or validation of others in inappropriate ways. Reading accounts of other men that realized a gay life was not for them was incredibly uplifting, and I gained much from their shared experiences. Tim Timmerman's book A Bigger World Yet: Faith, Brotherhood & Same Sex Needs engaged me in honesty with myself and others.

**Most helpful?**

Through personal counseling, honesty with myself and other men, discovering the real me, and

Journey Into Manhood—these were all factors in contributing to me being brave enough to explore the real me and to believe that I could change, that healing was possible and restoration was definitely possible. Most helpful were my therapist John Hinson, and Journey Into Manhood. Also Samson Society.

**Less helpful, or even harmful?**

Over-spiritualizing what was not a spiritual problem. Coercion from gay-identified men to "accept myself."

**Other benefits?**

I like me for the first time in my life. I feel more of a man than I ever have before, and I'm confident I'll stand up for my own rights as a man.

Frankly, I'd be dead today if I had not done the work required over time. I now have the passion to help other men who suffer in silence, shame, and self-abuse in many addictive forms. I will earn my master's degree in Clinical Mental Health Counseling soon, and obtain my Licensed Professional Counselor license. I live life openly. My former behavior does not label or identify me.

I'm proud to be well on the way of becoming the man that I believe I was meant to me; there's no greater joy or testosterone boost than that! I now have the confidence to experience the men's weekend by the ManKind Project (New Warrior Training Adventure) with men from any and all backgrounds, I never would have done this before engaging in being vulnerable to trust reparative therapy. Reparative therapy has *not* taken anything away from me; it has helped me *add* and *gain* what I needed. Autonomy is a beautiful thing, and a constitutional right.

# Tyler, 33, lives in Utah USA, Heterosexually Married, Latter-day Saint

| Major reduction in SSA *behaviors/ relationships* | Moderate reduction in same-sex *attractions* | Major increase in OSA *behaviors/ relationships* | Major increase in opposite-sex *attractions* | | | | | | | |
|---|---|---|---|---|---|---|---|---|---|---|

| Then | | | | | Now | | |
|---|---|---|---|---|---|---|---|
| *Exclusively homosexual* | Primarily homosexual but with incidental *heterosexual attractions* | Primarily homosexual but with significant *heterosexual attractions* | *About equally heterosexual and homosexual* | Primarily heterosexual but with significant *homosexual attractions* | Primarily heterosexual but with incidental *homosexual attractions* | *Exclusively heterosexual* |

**SSA "then"**  I never felt or identified as effeminate, but I certainly did not feel or identify with masculinity either. The vast majority of my friends were girls through elementary, middle and high school. I started viewing homosexual pornography at 14, and would struggle with that for years to come. I had enough heterosexual attraction that I felt tentatively okay with marrying a woman. After marriage, I struggled to find deep, meaningful physical connection with my wife. I eventually began to "act out" with other men, and this turned into frequent encounters with multiple partners. Pornography and Internet chat rooms became essential to coping with even the slightest degree of stress.

**Motivations**  I wanted marriage to a woman, I wanted a family, I wanted kids. I had all of those things and still felt so disconnected from who I was. This work helped me build a bridge from a place of disconnect to being able to enjoy the things I had worked for. I am religious; I believe the Book of Mormon to contain truth; I believe it was translated through the power of God; I believe my wife and I can be together as a family after death. I also believe, for me, continuing in a homosexual lifestyle would have put all the things I have worked for in jeopardy.

**SSA now**  Today, I am still very attracted to men, but it is different. I seek genuine, legitimate friendships with men instead of mere sexual gratification. Because of Journey into Manhood and other People Can Change initiatives, I strongly identify with and even celebrate my own masculinity. I have fantastic and meaningful physical relations with my wife. While I still occasionally relapse with pornography addiction, those times are outliers instead of the norm.

**What brought about change?**  I attended extensive counseling that was essential in being able to tear down the broken and unhealthy parts of my relationship with my parents and with many others in my life. It also gave me the opportunity and space to make a full disclosure to my spouse. I worked with my church leaders; their support and love for me was genuine and heartfelt.

**Most helpful?**  Journey into Manhood was a huge piece of my journey, as was Journey Beyond. Most helpful was having a place to express whatever I was afraid to express, and just be completely authentic and then seeing that I was still loved—I was, in fact, "valuable and good, just as I am."[11] Knowing I had other men who saw all the things I had kept hidden for so long, and not merely my attractions, but my misdeeds and my character flaws, and even after seeing all of this, they accepted me.

**Less helpful, or even harmful?**  Being told to "be true to myself" by friends who meant well in pushing me to leave my family and live a homosexual life. A media culture that idealizes and glorifies homosexuality, while mocking and ridiculing a person who has those feelings but chooses not to act on them.

**Any other benefits?**  I have experienced a substantial boost to my self-confidence, to my ability to communicate, and in my ability to lead. I work out at the gym and take care of my physical body, not as a thing of vanity, but because I am worth taking that time for. I have a greater, more fulfilling relationship with my spouse, with my kids, with my parents, and with numerous friends and mentors.

---

[11] Journey Into Manhood program. See also http://www.peoplecanchange.com/change/notshame.php

# Ronald, 50, lives in California USA, Single, Christian

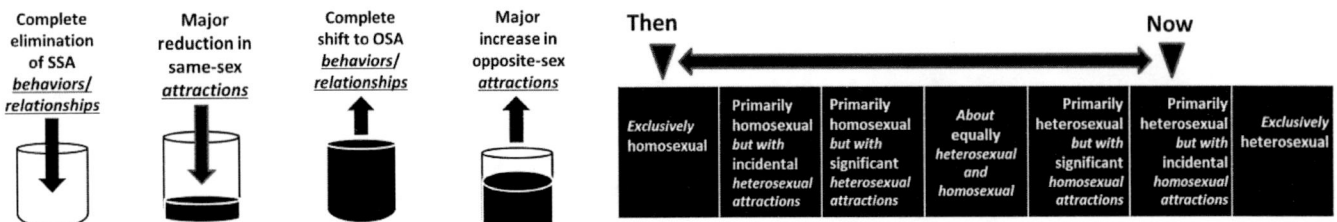

**SSA "then"**

I was a self-affirmed, out-of-the-closet, fully identified gay man. I was in a relationship with another man for 18 years. I had absolutely no heterosexual desire. By the world's standards, I was moderately successful. We owned a house, had two cars and many friends. Yet deep down inside I was miserable. I was very sexually active with many partners. And I felt complete empty.

**Motivations**

After 18 years of living the gay lifestyle, I had come to an end of myself. I did not like anything about who I was and where I was going. I grew up in a Christian household and decided that I would give God one more chance. I had tried everything else in order to make myself feel better and more connected. Nothing worked. It was in a life of submission to the Lordship of Jesus Christ that I found my answer. He is what motivates me to live the life I live now. I often say that the opposite of homosexuality is not heterosexuality, it is holiness. It is living a life based on biblical principles, honoring God and serving Jesus and other people.

**SSA now**

Today I am happily celibate. I just started dating a very nice young woman. My same-sex attractions have depleted to the point where they are almost non-existent. While I do experience attractions to other men on occasion, they are more of a desire to compare myself or to get to know the other man relationally, not sexually.

**What brought about change?**

I found a ministry in San Rafael, California that offered help to those who struggled with same-sex attractions. I left my partner, my house, my job and moved to San Rafael to become part of a live-in ministry. There, I learned the underlying roots of why I was attracted to my own gender. I pushed through the initial desire to have sex and sought out ways to enjoy the relational company of other men. As I gained friends and began to serve in my church and community, my attractions began to diminish. Little by little, with the help of a professional therapist, a really good pastor and people who truly cared about me, my attitude, behaviors and the way I thought about myself and others began to change.

**Most helpful?**

My relationship with God through Jesus Christ. Other Christian men and women to walk with me and hold me accountable. The desire for transformation, which included my own attitude and willingness to stick with it even when it was uncomfortable, scary or made me mad.

**Less helpful, or even harmful?**

Nothing.

**Any other benefits?**

Absolutely! I am no longer a man searching for something to fill and satisfy. I have found that in my relationship with Christ. I have a deep and true sense of who I am, where I have come from and where I am going. Every day is part of a new journey, with each day bringing its own difficulties, trials, and joys. I no longer go on the hunt for sexual exploits or conquests. Instead, I seek out positive, affirming relationships with both men and women that are relationally appropriate and still challenging.

# Charles David, 54, lives in South Africa, Single, Christian (Reformed Christian)

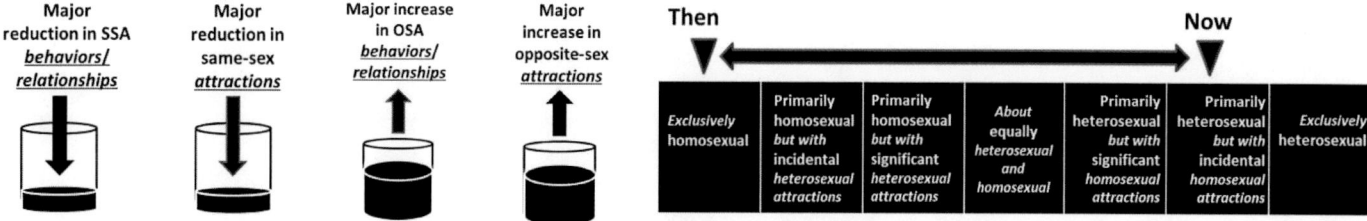

| | | Then ◄─────────────────────────► Now | | | | | |
|---|---|---|---|---|---|---|---|
| Major reduction in SSA *behaviors/ relationships* | Major reduction in same-sex *attractions* | Major increase in OSA *behaviors/ relationships* | Major increase in opposite-sex *attractions* | | | | |

**SSA "then"**

My SSA was strong and self-identified at a young age, which was traumatic and confusing for me, leading me to believe that change was not possible. While in the gay scene, I was in a five-year relationship, and even though I had multiple partners I never considered myself promiscuous.

**Motivations**

I can and never could reconcile my physical, emotional, moral and spiritual values, with one of an active homosexual lifestyle or orientation. My spirituality, faith, my relationship with and devotion to God are all vital for me. Homosexuality is a "dead-end" for me.

**SSA now**

My same-sex attractions have certainly diminished over time, as I actively avoided and completely abstained from sexual encounters and have not fed myself with gay porn, fantasy or compulsive masturbation. There are certain women who I find very attractive, in the sense of an inner natural beauty, and over time, having gotten to know them better, a courtship could develop. I feel I could get married. Yes, I would like a wife and children. However, this is not a major agenda item. I'm happy and content being single and celibate at the moment.

**What brought about change?**

I came out of the gay scene and lifestyle, losing many friends as a result. It was lonely at times, but worth it. I allowed my SSA to be de-sensitized and minimized with healthy, non-erotic male friendships and gym buddies. I realized I *am* heterosexual and already had all the traits, characteristics and potential of the men I previously sexualized. I *am* a man among men! I opened myself up to female friendships. Telling myself and others the truth set me free. I put off old thought patterns and replaced them with a new mindset. Knowing and applying principles I read and certain teachings I learned was extremely beneficial. Mere information became *personal conviction*. I have come to know myself, and I now make myself known to others.

**Most helpful?**

Honest and transparent one-on-one pastoral counseling over an extended period of time. It was exacting and sometimes very demoralizing, but I pushed through, and am where I am today. There are however still minor scars—remnants and residues from my active gay past that may never go away. Making new, quality friends and hearing and reading personal testimonies of others who had changed were also very helpful.

I became involved in my local church community and gave out to others. I also finally understood the big difference between same-sex attractions as opposed to same-sex actions. The one is your choice—the other not! Also important was group interaction on forums such as <u>People Can Change</u>, Ex-Gay Discussion Board and <u>Setting Captives Free</u>—knowing you're not alone and that there are concerned and caring brothers out there.

**Less helpful, or even harmful?**

Some of the questionable teachings, devices and methods that were used as I pursued the pathway to transformation. I just tested and examined everything—and held onto what is good and true and disregard the rest.

**Any other benefits?**

Life-changing!

**Alan,** 53, lives in Texas USA, Heterosexually Married, Catholic

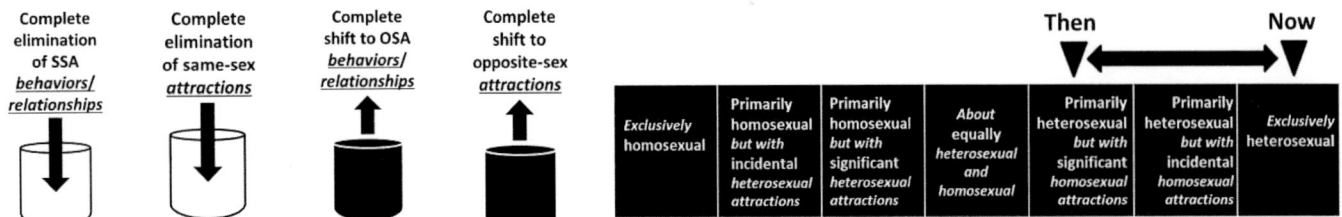

| **Motivations** | What motivated me was, first, the fact that acting on my homosexual attractions is not compatible with my religious beliefs. Second, acting on them would destroy my relationship with my wife, whom I dearly love. I could not bear to inflict that kind of hurt and pain on her and my young children. |
|---|---|
| **SSA now** | I am now exclusively opposite-sex attracted, to the point that heterosexual pornography has been an issue for me. |
| **What brought about change?** | Deep emotional release work, self-primal therapy, 12 Step groups, experiential retreats, past reality integration therapy, centering prayer. Deep process release support groups (Anne Wilson Schaef's work). |
| **Most helpful?** | Deep work of the type mentioned above. |
| **Less helpful, or even harmful?** | Exodus type of support groups. Although I only went a few times, I knew that singing hymns and praying, with no deep work, would not be for me.<br><br>Deep work is very difficult at times, but I have never been happier in my life. Nothing negative has ever come of it. |
| **Any other benefits?** | Self-esteem increase. Masculinity increase. |

# Markus, 51, lives in Germany. Heterosexually Married, Catholic

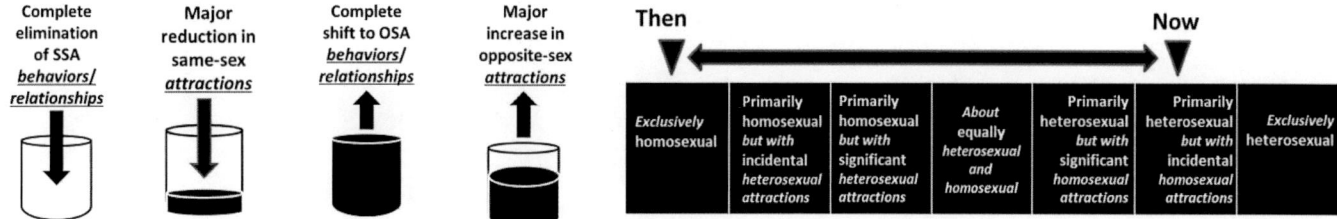

**SSA "then"**

I had over 300 sexual contacts with other men I did not really know. I met them in gay saunas, gay bars or in parks. I lived also in a relationship with a boyfriend for one year, and with another for five years. I identified myself as a gay man because I never heard about any chance to change the orientation. But I never felt good in that lifestyle. I hated myself, I hated how I looked, and I thought I needed another man to rescue me out of these feelings.

**Motivations**

For me, homosexuality was a way to deal with my self-hatred. From early childhood, I never could be in relationship with other boys or men without thinking, I am wrong or I am not as attractive as other guys. In kindergarten, I found that fantasizing about boys who are more popular than me would reduce my inner stress. This was the source of my homosexual feelings. Despite hundreds of sexual contacts with men, none of them met my inner needs nor helped to reduce the self-hatred. I even tried to commit suicide.

**SSA now**

In therapy I found a way to work through my fears of other man and through my self-hatred. The more I worked through the trauma behind all of this, the more feelings of self-acceptance and inner peace emerged and increased. This was also true in my relationships with men. When this happened, my homosexual attractions decreased step by step, and heterosexual feelings arose. Today I have been married to my wife since 1991, and we have three kids. I am attracted to my wife and to other women.

Sometimes when I am stressed or have to face a lot of challenges, I sense that I lose my inner stability and identity. Sometimes then I feel an attraction toward strong men, where I tell myself that they handle their life easily. But this attraction is not very strong now, and I don't need to look for sex with a man.

**What brought about change?**

I have used trauma therapy and body work to come out of the shame and the trauma that stood behind my self-hatred. Also I used sessions of Gestalt and transaction analysis. But trauma therapy and a body-oriented therapy helped me most.

**Most helpful?**

Counseling and therapy

**Less helpful, or even harmful?**

Everything was helpful on my way to understand myself better. There was nothing harmful.

**Any other benefits?**

There are a lot of benefits. The focus of the therapy never was the sexual attraction towards men. My therapist was focused on my stress with men, my fears in relationships, my depression, and my self-hatred. Today I am more secure in relationships with men and women. I have more self-esteem. I feel more masculine. I am in freedom with other men. I don't feel shame or fear of other man. I have more boundaries and I can set healthy boundaries in my relationships.

# "Monty," 24, lives in New York USA, Single, Jewish

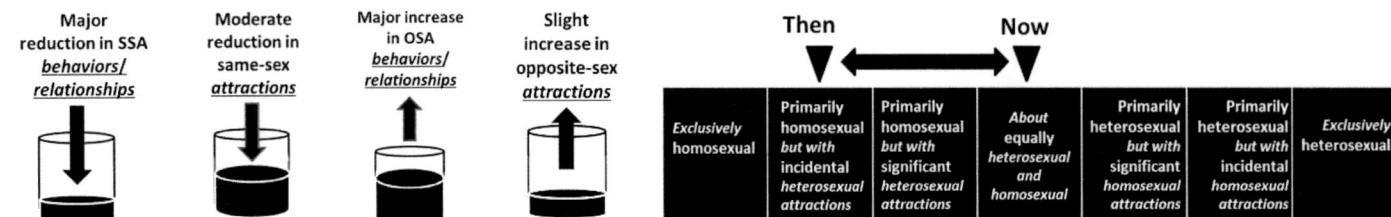

| | | |
|---|---|---|
| Major reduction in SSA *behaviors/relationships* | Moderate reduction in same-sex *attractions* | Major increase in OSA *behaviors/relationships* | Slight increase in opposite-sex *attractions* |

**Then** ⟷ **Now**

| Exclusively homosexual | Primarily homosexual *but with incidental heterosexual attractions* | Primarily homosexual *but with significant heterosexual attractions* | About equally *heterosexual and homosexual* | Primarily heterosexual *but with significant homosexual attractions* | Primarily heterosexual *but with incidental homosexual attractions* | Exclusively heterosexual |

**SSA "then"**

I was depressed, compulsive, angry, hyper-sexual and avoidant. I was closeted and shamed. I was suicidal. I was outed and shamed more. I wanted to die.

**Motivations**

My same-sex attractions did not resonate with the way I wanted to live my life. Part of the motivation was spiritual. Part of it was societal. But mainly, homosexuality just wasn't working for me.

**SSA now**

I'm so much healthier mentally, spiritually and physically. There are men I'm attracted to but I am not controlled by those attractions. I have deep meaningful connections with men, both gay and straight, that are completely platonic. I am much more attracted to women, though I was always sexually attracted to them. I do feel however that I am in a space to be in a romantic relationship now, where that wasn't the case before.

**What brought about change?**

Went to counseling by a licensed therapist in Israel. Experiential workshops. Lots of time and patience. Since beginning my work, I have experienced a reduction in SSA, though it is in direct relationship to how disciplined I am to align myself with the values I deem appropriate. The more I work, the more the reduction. If I sit around and don't put effort into my own personal work and development, I slip back into old destructive patterns, both sexual and not.

**Most helpful?**

Call of the Shofar. Journey Beyond. My therapist.

**Less helpful, or even harmful?**

I can't think of anything.

**Final comments?**

Of course I was working on myself overall, not just my sexuality. I recognize that change efforts aren't for everyone. My gay friends are happy with their choices, as are my SSA friends. Can everyone change? I haven't the slightest clue. But is change possible for some? Definitely. It is also imperative that it doesn't become a shaming experience.

# "Yaakov," 37, lives in California USA, Single, Jewish

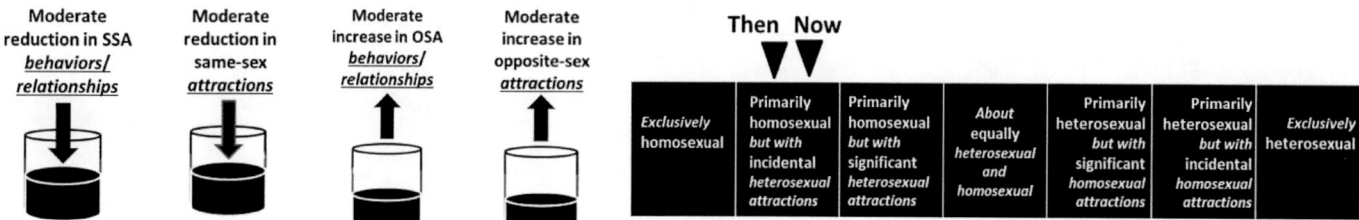

| | | | | | |
|---|---|---|---|---|---|
| Moderate reduction in SSA *behaviors/ relationships* | Moderate reduction in same-sex *attractions* | Moderate increase in OSA *behaviors/ relationships* | Moderate increase in opposite-sex *attractions* | **Then Now** | |

| *Exclusively homosexual* | Primarily homosexual *but with incidental heterosexual attractions* | Primarily homosexual *but with significant heterosexual attractions* | *About equally heterosexual and homosexual* | Primarily heterosexual *but with significant homosexual attractions* | Primarily heterosexual *but with incidental homosexual attractions* | *Exclusively heterosexual* |

**SSA "then"**

SSA was a strong feeling, but something I never articulated or acted on (outside of fantasy during masturbation). At the time, I wanted to believe the feelings would just go away if I ignored them, and I felt extremely anxious about those feelings when they came up. Over time, I became somewhat hopeless that the feelings would ever resolve, and I felt like all options available to me were unattractive. I had trouble sleeping, and often felt extremely down.

**Motivations**

Desire for a traditional family structure. Lack of interest in a gay lifestyle.

**SSA now**

My sexual behavior is mostly unchanged (I never was sexually active), though I tend to masturbate less. My same-sex attraction is modestly diminished, but far more importantly, I am comfortable with that as a part of who I am. I am open about it with my friends and have mostly found a way to get those needs for intimacy met with men through non-sexual outlets. This mostly resolves my conflict, and I have been able to pursue dating women with more confidence and openness. It has resulted in a modestly increased attraction to women sexually, and much more desire for connection with a woman romantically.

**What brought about change?**

Counseling (through a JONAH-recommended therapist), Journey Into Manhood/People Can Change, building a community of men for support. These things, combined, resulted in much more personal acceptance and self-love. I would not be anywhere near as satisfied without them.

**Most helpful?**

Counseling, but each piece was crucial.

**Less helpful, or even harmful?**

I have had no negative effects from my change efforts. Just the opposite. I considered both change and gay-affirmative options to be a difficult challenge with potential risks. Doing nothing wasn't an option for me any longer, but gay-affirmation seemed much more radical and permanent. I considered the change option to be more measured and reversible if it didn't work for me.

**Any other benefits?**

Massive improvements in life outlook, self-acceptance, sense of masculinity, reduction in anxiety.

# Chuck, 56, lives in Florida USA, Heterosexually married, Non-religious

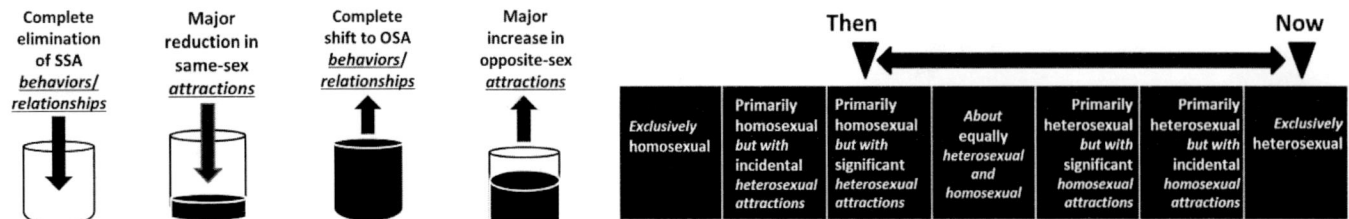

| | | | | | | |
|---|---|---|---|---|---|---|
| Complete elimination of SSA *behaviors/ relationships* | Major reduction in same-sex *attractions* | Complete shift to OSA *behaviors/ relationships* | Major increase in opposite-sex *attractions* | | Then | Now |

| Exclusively homosexual | Primarily homosexual *but with incidental heterosexual attractions* | Primarily homosexual *but with significant heterosexual attractions* | *About equally heterosexual and homosexual* | Primarily heterosexual *but with significant homosexual attractions* | Primarily heterosexual *but with incidental homosexual attractions* | Exclusively heterosexual |

**SSA "then"**

I was a married man ("closeted" or so I believed), with children, who was acting out my SSA daily in the form of sexual encounters, web-camming, and use of gay pornography. I was into group sex, S&M, the drug scene, one-on-one encounters, bath houses, and used different social media to fulfill my desires. I was attracted to my wife, but more motivated to seek sexual gratification from men. This behavior spanned a 10-year period, until I learned I had choices and realized the behavior was not making me happy, just depressed and isolated from real friendships that I had abandoned. Over that 10-year span, I likely had sexual relations with over 1,000 men.

**Motivations**

I began to understand that what I was really seeking was non-sexual affirmation from the world of men. Sexual gratification never filled the underlying void. I felt deep in my core that I was not homosexual; rather, I had sexualized those male qualities I judged I never possessed, including sports ability, a muscular physique and other masculine physical qualities, strength of character, and more—all things that I deemed different from me.

I had strong attraction to women, both emotionally and sexually. With men, it was all physical and never emotional. I came to realize that I would never be "enough" for any man, nor would they be for me. Only the feminine could provide me with complementary, not competitive, strength and love.

**SSA now**

Every aspect of my life is better. I am more grounded, mature, satisfied with myself, easier to get along with, able to make choices, and set clear boundaries. My marriage is better than I could have dreamed, and my wife is now my best friend. We can discuss issues and concerns openly without leading to resentment, even when we do not agree. My children know about my struggles, and this has only improved our relationships. I own my masculinity. I also know what I do not possess in terms of those attributes that I used to sexualize. I have learned through many experiential processes that I am fully masculine, regardless. I am still working to be a better person, more generous and authentic.

**What brought about change?**

I started with local counseling and a support group for sexual addiction and was open about my sexuality at the time. I attended a 12 Step support group meeting (Sex Addicts Anonymous) weekly and worked the steps. I read books on homosexuality, coming out, etc., but did not feel they fit me accurately in any way. I lucked onto a book about reparative therapy by Joseph Nicolosi and began to resonate with his writings and theories. I sought out real reparative therapy and pursued it aggressively.

I attended Journey Into Manhood, which completely improved my self-esteem and concept of sexuality, due to the psychodramtic processes I experienced, but also because of the safe community of non-sexual male friendships I developed. I lost all shame for any prior behaviors and began to openly discuss my transformation with others who were interested. I have returned the favor by staffing subsequent weekends for Journey Into Manhood. I attended an advanced experiential learning weekend called Journey Beyond that further solidified my sense of mature masculinity, and I have staffed that weekend subsequently.

I attended <u>The Noble Man</u>, an experiential weekend run by women, who helped me stop transferring my relationship with my mother onto my wife and most women I knew. I attended the <u>New Warrior Training Adventure</u>, which taught me how to communicate openly with men of all faiths and sexualities. I developed confidence to be the man I was intended to be. I meet with my <u>ManKind Project </u>(New Warrior) brothers weekly, to continue healthy relationships with salient, encouraging men. They are straight, bi, and gay, and I love and trust each one with some of the most private and intimate details of my life.

I am keenly aware that what has worked for me to change my sexual behaviors and desires is not appropriate for everyone, but it was my personal choice to change my thoughts and behaviors. I have no religious orientation, so I am not motivated by any orthodoxy of any kind. I do this work for myself.

**Most helpful?**  Each experience of my journey has filled a different aspect of my change in primary sexuality. If I had to pick two, they would be the <u>People Can Change </u>experiential weekend trainings like <u>Journey Into Manhood </u>and <u>Journey Beyond</u>, and therapy with a properly trained reparative therapist.

**Less helpful, or even harmful?**  Some aspects of my experience with the <u>New Warrior Training Adventure </u>have been wounding, since many men do not believe I can change my sexual orientation. This has resulted in my own pull-back from their training weekends and advanced-level staff trainings.

**Any other benefits?**  I have never been more grounded and mature in my life.

**Final comment?**  My caution is that this work may not work for most. But it remains my right to choose how to live my life without persecution and ridicule. I have friends who tried to change but didn't make it. I always tell them that all I ever want for them is to be happy inside, no matter what their sexual orientation is. I cannot convince anyone to try my way. It has to be an internal, self-motivated desire. Where I see sadness and lack of satisfaction in life is with men—straight, gay, SSA or whatever—who have untreated mental disorders or who cannot be happy with their choices. Those men will never find joy and freedom, no matter what sexual orientation they have.

# Stephen, 42, lives in Texas USA, Heterosexually Married, Christian (Church of Christ)

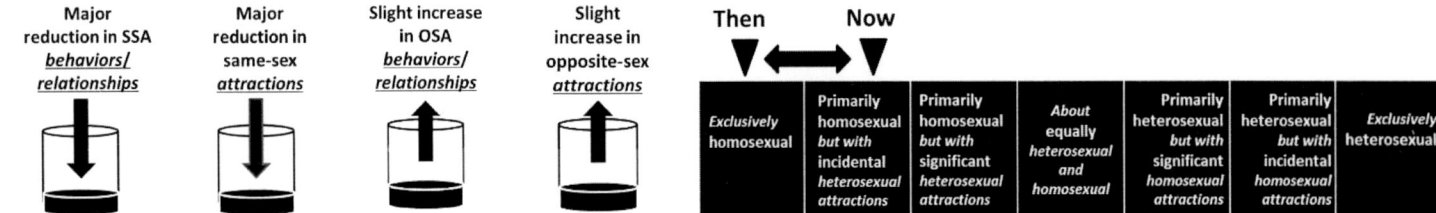

**SSA "then"**

I was cruising pornography stores and public parks during the height of my SSA, nearly every day and sometimes multiple times a day. I would guess over 400 homosexual interactions, primarily mutual masturbation. I spent lots of money and time in these nasty places, hiding from the hetero world to escape into a homosexual world. Acting out with another male brought release from the stress of remaining in the closet and not revealing these unwanted SSA feelings to friends and family.

**Motivations**

Through the faith instilled from my parents and the overall conviction of wanting to spend my eternal home in Heaven, I recognize homosexuality as a sin. The counseling, support groups, personal relationships, my wife and self-help methods (books, testimonies, retreats, conferences), a deeper faith, maturity in age and the desire to honor my marriage vows, I hold fast to the truths proclaimed by God who gave His only Son for my transgressions.

**SSA now**

Today I have a degree of sexual sobriety that I once thought was impossible to achieve. True, my SSA feelings are still there, but they are turned over more towards my Father in Heaven, casting my anxieties on Him. Also, with a greater understanding of grace, I have been able to let go if the insatiable need to "act out" sexually. I have learned tools to dissolve SSA feelings and work within boundaries of healthy friendships...not sexcapades.

**What brought about change?**

Grace from God and learning to forgive myself, accepting that he does love me. Grace from my wife and friends. Guidance from elders in my church. Guidance from fellow strugglers who also do not want SSA. Celebrate Recovery. Sexaholics Anonymous.

**Most helpful?**

My counselor, and non-judgmental, grace-driven brothers in Christ.

**Less helpful, or even harmful?**

A pastor who betrayed homosexual boundaries with me. It put a sting in my faith that has taken years to recover from.

**Any other benefits?**

Better boundaries with male friendships. Re-creating a healthy marriage. Friends who know my SSA feelings and are not afraid to be around me.

# Blake, 59, lives in California USA, Heterosexually Married, Latter-day Saint

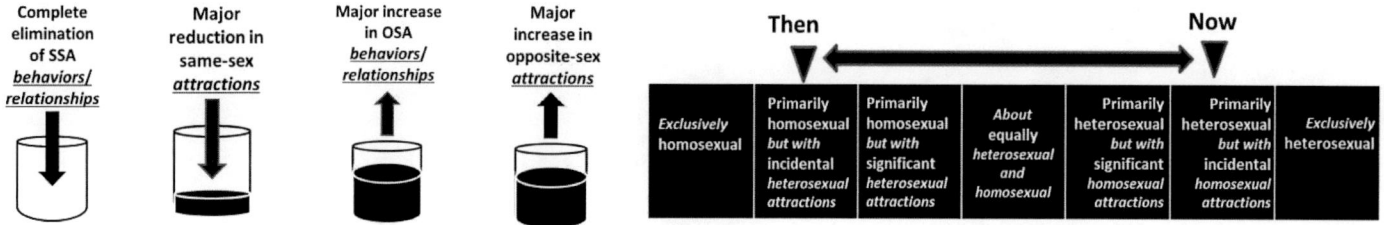

**SSA "then"**

I was closeted and repressed, living in mortal fear of being found out. Masturbation was almost constant. I was isolated from everyone. I didn't go into the gay community because that was not how I lived. My participation in the straight life was a joke and a lie. I believed that if I did "as-if living," it would go away. It didn't. Shame and isolation were how I lived, all of the time craving male sexual contact. I contemplated suicide often and attempted once. I wanted so much for it to go away so that I could live my religion and have a family like everyone else. It was a horrible way to live.

**Motivations**

I did not want to live like that. In my opinion, the day I decided not to act on my same-sex attractions, I made a life-and-death decision, given my age and the number of gay men in my age group who died of AIDS before the improvements in medications. I wanted to be a husband and father and I wanted to live in conformity with my religious beliefs. I craved male sexual contact 24 hours a day, seven days a week. I controlled myself all day, just to dream about it at night. I hated living like that. My life was consumed in shame and self-loathing, and I lived in constant fear that people would find out what I felt. I just plain wanted it to go away and not come back.

**SSA now**

Over time I have experienced an almost complete elimination of my same-sex feelings. My constant craving went away. The dreams went away. I have almost NO sexual attractions to men. I do experience memories of past feelings and experiences, but I have no desire to have sex with men most of the time.

My view of men has changed completely and so has my view of women. I have an amazing marriage to a wonderful woman. I am respected by a lot of straight men who couldn't imagine where I was 30 years ago. I used to view gay porn; I don't anymore. I used to just crave inappropriate relationships with men; now I have healthy relationships with men and I am respected as one of them. I have a great sex life with my current wife. My first marriage was a disaster and would have been without regard to my SSA. Because of my Journey Beyond experience, I find myself attracted to women that I see walking down the street or in meetings. I love experiencing the feelings, and I embrace the opportunity to have sexual desires for many attractive women. This came about directly because of Journey Beyond.

**What brought about change?**

Around 25 years ago I attended my first ex-gay ministry meeting. That began a journey. I attended the meetings and read everything I could get my hands on. That was a period of intense learning. During that time I had a really good therapist who began helping me process my traumas, and the support of a bishop in my church who offered amazing support and help through the process. He was my rock, my support, and my strength. I learned what real love between men was supposed to look like.

1. My own motivation and commitment to the process is primary.

2. My faith in God gave me the strength to keep going when my own commitment failed.

3. A strong support system of strong, healthy men who love and accept me for who I am.

4. Excellent counseling to help me process my many traumas.

5. Participating in experiential retreats, whether they focused on SSA or not.

6. Staffing experiential retreats that focus on SSA.

7. <u>12 Step</u> programs.

8. I read a lot of good, helpful books.

9. <u>Cognitive Behavioral Therapy</u> that I did using a book that helped me change my thoughts and attitudes.

**Most helpful?** My first staffing of <u>Journey Into Manhood</u> pretty much put the nail in the coffin of my desires to have sex with men. My attractions to women can tie back directly to processes at <u>Journey Beyond</u>. The help that I received from a bishop 20 years ago did the most. It was, in my opinion, miraculous. I can never repay what he did for me.

**Less helpful, or even harmful?** I didn't have any negative experiences in my change efforts. But I'm sure if I had followed the gay-affirming path when I was making my life decisions, the most likely scenario is that I would be dead from AIDS now.

Also less helpful: Therapists who had no business trying to help me. Some had no respect for my therapeutic goals; i.e., reduction of SSA feelings and increase in OSA feelings.

**Any other benefits?** My self-esteem has increased dramatically, and I have a strongly increased inner sense of masculinity to the point that other men sense it and treat me completely differently than they used to. Strangely enough, my <u>Journey Into Manhood</u> weekend cured a long-standing sugar addiction, and I lost 15 pounds as a direct result of doing the underlying work revealed to me on my JiM weekend. I have been able to take out many life traumas, examine them, and put them where they belong so that they no longer have control over my life.

My view of men and women has completely changed. I have learned to love men for what they are and have no desire to have sex with them. I used to view most women as bitches out to manipulate and control me. I no longer see women like that. <u>Journey Beyond</u> did more to help me with that than anything else that I did. I have a deep sense of love and compassion for people, viewing them as sons and daughters of a loving Heavenly Father rather than in any negative light. When I think back on how much I have changed over the last 30 years, it blows me away. There is almost nothing about me that is what I was like 30 years ago. I love every change.

# Benjamin, 37, lives in California USA, Single, Christian

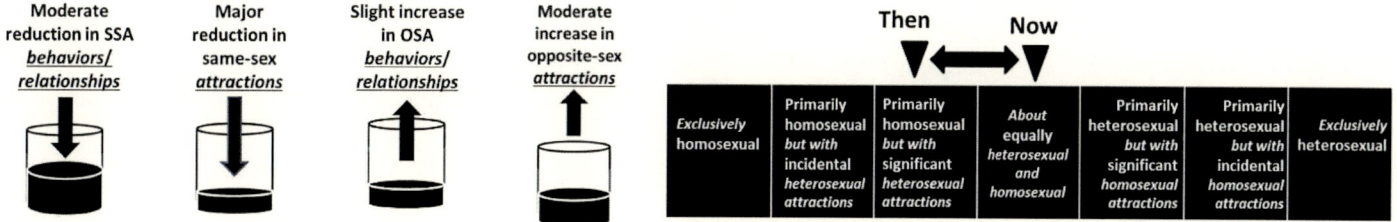

**SSA "then"**

At the strongest point, I looked at pornography basically daily and drank quite a bit to try and ease the sense of conflict and hopelessness I was feeling. I found myself participating in sexual relationships that I really did not feel comfortable with, which had no wholesome emotional bond and left me feeling empty and degraded afterwards. But I felt so desperate for male connection that I participated anyway. I would see a guy and become obsessed with him. I would feel desperate to connect. I wanted him to know me, be close to me and love me.

**Motivations**

At first it was mainly my religious beliefs, although I never felt like taking on an identity as gay would be an authentic expression of who I am. As I have done more personal work on the emotions and beliefs that underlie my attractions, I have felt more and more that a gay identity does not express who I truly am. My religious beliefs still guide me, but in the area of sexuality and identity, I am guided more by a growing sense of grounded identity, which causes those former attractions to fade away or alter in their nature.

**SSA now**

My sexual attractions to guys are far less than they used to be. They happen less often and are not as strong. I still find men attractive, but the desires are primarily desires to be friends, to get to know each other, to somehow become more like what I see in him. There's not nearly as much of that same needy, clingy desperate feeling. I find that my brotherly male friendships bring an incredible sense of joy and peace into my life. Sexual connection or exclusive relationship scenarios fade in the light of the joy I feel with my brothers.

I find myself approaching women as a strong, assertive, grounded male. Some of my old female friends can't handle it very well because they are used to the old me, who I view now as having been a very weak and clingy little boy who would follow girls around because it felt comfortable. Now I feel my own power as a male and carry more confidence. I respect women without sacrificing parts of myself. It's a good feeling. It makes women more appealing. I don't plan on having sex with a woman unless I marry her first. But that is becoming more and more desirable to me.

**What brought about change**

I have done most of my work on experiential weekends such as the Journey Into Manhood and Adventure In Manhood weekends, which focus on same-sex attraction issues, and the Living From the Heart weekends and New Warrior Training Adventure, which allow space for men to work on issues around their sexuality and the emotions that influence them. I also did a five-month program called Living Waters, which is more of a spiritually based Christian program. My journey has also been greatly influenced by speakers at an SSA group I attend as well as online courses offered by therapists. My life coach also specializes in same-sex attractions.

**Most helpful**

Journey Into Manhood and the support groups associated with it have been by far the most helpful.

**Less helpful, or even harmful**

My experiences with a therapist who told me I was born gay were, in my opinion, harmful. I would go to this therapist with relative peace of mind, not even planning on doing work related to my same-sex attractions. He kept steering the conversation to same-sex attractions. I would leave incredibly agitated, feeling like I hadn't been heard out. He simply wrote off the parts of my experiences that could not be explained in the scenario he was trying to convince me of: that people are born gay and there was nothing that could change sexual attractions. This was after I had already experienced some changes in my attractions. He taught me just how damaging it can be when a therapist pushes an agenda onto his client. It was as if I didn't matter as a person.

**Other benefits?**  I'm much more confident. I love myself more. I'm more in touch with my emotions. I have deeper, more fulfilling friendships with others. I have a better sense of what I want in life and am able to assert myself towards it. I have many more tools available to me now so that when the ups and downs of life come, I am able to gauge what is going on inside me. I can identify my needs and determine ways to meet them that are in line with my beliefs.

# Carmine, 69, lives in Indiana USA, Single, Catholic

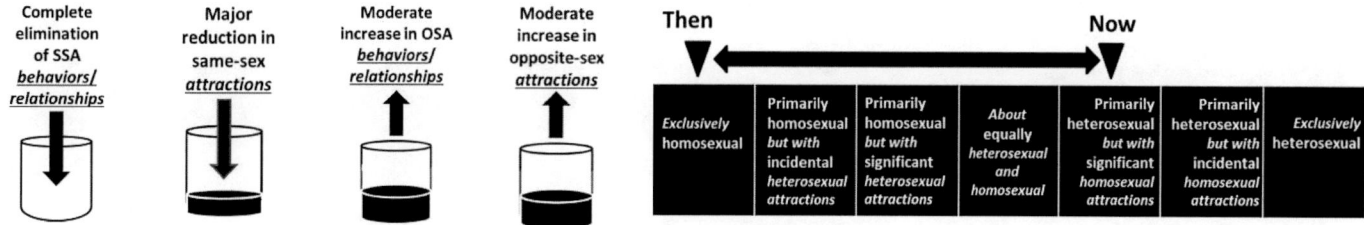

| | Complete elimination of SSA *behaviors/ relationships* | Major reduction in same-sex *attractions* | Moderate increase in OSA *behaviors/ relationships* | Moderate increase in opposite-sex *attractions* |
|---|---|---|---|---|

**SSA "then"**
My homosexual feelings were "out of control." To put it simply, I was a homosexual sex addict. Although well closeted, I frequently acted out with pornography and even once had anonymous sex with someone I met in a gay bar. I thought that if I just accepted the reality that I was gay my acting out would decrease. However, I found that identifying as gay did not sit well with who I really felt I was inside. I felt that I was in constant turmoil, living a lie no matter which way I turned.

**Motivations**
Primarily, my religious beliefs. While my religion does not condemn the orientation itself, it does say that the actions are sinful. My attractions were so strong that I frequently compulsively acted out my feelings, and that created a lot of inner conflict for me. I sought the help of <u>People Can Change</u> to reduce or eliminate my attractions.

**SSA now**
While my homosexual attractions have not completed disappeared, the have diminished quite significantly. Also, although I still have some attractions, my interest or desire for the sexual activity has almost completely evaporated. Also, I frequently catch myself "checking out" some attractive females despite the fact that I have no intentions of pursuing a heterosexual relationship. I am still working through some other issues I have around women that would hamper a healthy heterosexual relationship.

My main focus has not been to increase my heterosexual behavior (which, outside of marriage, my religion also considers sinful) but to live a healthy celibate life.

**What brought about change?**
The biggest and most significant step I took was to make a <u>Journey Into Manhood</u> weekend back in 2006. All my other efforts (<u>Sex Addicts Anonymous</u>, <u>Adult Children of Alcoholics</u>, psychological counseling) helped very little or not at all. Journey Into Manhood was a real watershed in my life.

**Most helpful?**
<u>Journey Into Manhood</u> and a <u>follow-up telephone group</u>.

**Less helpful, or even harmful?**
Other supports were somewhat helpful for a while, but their effects always fizzled out. But I have not experienced any negative effects. Had I kept doing what I was doing, I would have been one miserable man, if not a dead one.

**Any other benefits?**
I must say that I have never been happier in my life. While still falling short in self-esteem, I feel good about myself and about who I am. There is still work to do, but I feel that I have the tools to do it.

**Final comments?**
Pursuing change is not for everyone. But those of us who are interested in doing so should have the right to do so. Since my motivation is primarily religious, I think my right is ultimately grounded in freedom of religion. If people like me are prevented from seeking freedom from a life of inner conflict and turmoil, we would be denied our right to pursue happiness.

**Sean,** 60, lives in Arizona USA, Single, Catholic

| Complete elimination of SSA *behaviors/ relationships* | Complete elimination of same-sex *attractions* | Major increase in OSA *behaviors/ relationships* | Complete shift to opposite-sex *attractions* | **Then** | | | | | | **Now** |
|---|---|---|---|---|---|---|---|---|---|---|

| *Exclusively homosexual* | Primarily homosexual *but with incidental heterosexual attractions* | Primarily homosexual *but with significant heterosexual attractions* | About equally *heterosexual and homosexual* | Primarily heterosexual *but with significant homosexual attractions* | Primarily heterosexual *but with incidental homosexual attractions* | *Exclusively heterosexual* |
|---|---|---|---|---|---|---|

**SSA "then"**  When my SSA was strongest, I lived a secret gay life. There was excitement over new sexual encounters, but even before I went through these acts I would regret it already, and ask myself, "Why am I doing this?" Then afterwards I would regret it even more. It was like drug addiction. It never felt good afterwards, but I felt driven to keep trying to satisfy the drives.

**Motivations**  Having lived the gay life for many years, I was struck by the pointlessness of it all and wondering how will this all end? I never felt like I was truly "me." I felt a disconnection from the community of men.

**SSA now**  My SSA is now gone. I have no desire to have sex with men. I am strongly attracted to having sex with women and look forward to it with great excitement. However, I am not sexually active. I am waiting for that one special woman to marry.

**What brought about change?**  I started therapy in March 2008. I was very motivated to change, so my progress was rapid. I also attended a weekend called Journey Into Manhood that really helped me deal with the issues that led up to my SSA.

**Most helpful?**  Counseling was most instrumental in addressing a lot of my contributing issues. The New Warrior Training Adventure and a process about my issues with women was exhilarating and liberating. An experiential weekend called The Noble Man was also very helpful in relating to women.

**Less helpful, or even harmful?**  I never experienced anything harmful. I think I would be in more danger if I never had any help in dealing with these unwanted sexual attractions. I am grateful I had that choice.

**Any other benefits?**  Improvements in my self-esteem. I've made many friends, which were few in number before my therapy. I also am more assertive. If I am ever hurt by others, I deal with it in the moment. I also feel a part of the community of men now instead of feeling alienated from them.

# "Rob," 47, lives in California USA, Heterosexually Married, Catholic

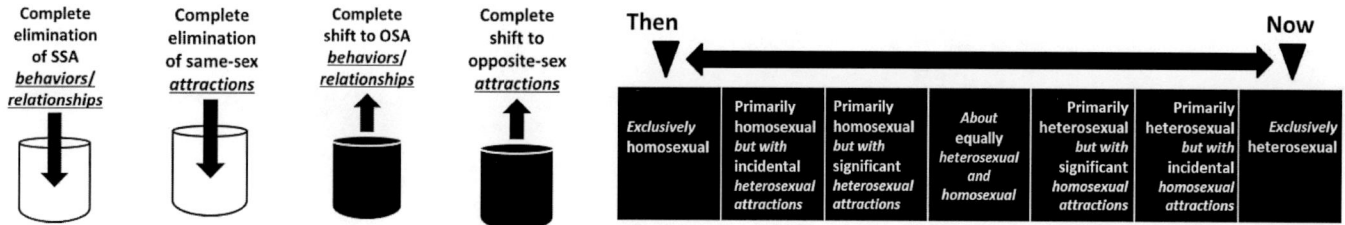

**SSA "then"**

Before, I was exclusively SSA. It seemed like my blood literally boiled with SSA lust. I had no physical or romantic attraction to women. I never acted on my desires, although I came close. It felt like it wasn't really me. And the closer I got to being sexual with a man, the sadder I became.

**Motivations**

I felt it was in conflict with my authentic self. It didn't make sense to me that God would create me to be gay. But I didn't know change was possible, and if it was, I was sure it wouldn't work for me!

**SSA now**

My same-sex needs now are fulfilled by affirmation, affiliation and platonic relationships with men. Men cannot give me what women can, and vice versa. I know now how to get my needs met by both genders without being incongruent with who I am as a man.

**What brought about change?**

Initially, I tried praying, dating women, white knuckling it—nothing worked. After I entered reparative therapy, I began discovering events in my past and patterns in my behavior that fueled my SSA. Slowly, with much time and effort, I felt shifts in my feelings, attractions and even my happiness.

Eventually, men faded into the background and women began to come into the forefront of my attractions. I began dating women again, with much different results. I eventually felt the desire to marry. I found a beautiful woman who knows everything about me and married her! Soon we will celebrate our eighth wedding anniversary. It keeps getting better every year. This from a guy who wasn't even comfortable holding a woman's hand!

**Most helpful?**

Counseling and Journey Into Manhood weekends. Counseling was critical, but experiential-healing work took it all to a new level!

**Less helpful, or even harmful?**

Denial and white knuckling. Living a double life.

**Any other benefits?**

Self-esteem and happiness both increased.

# "Eli," 60, lives in Israel, Heterosexually Married, Jewish

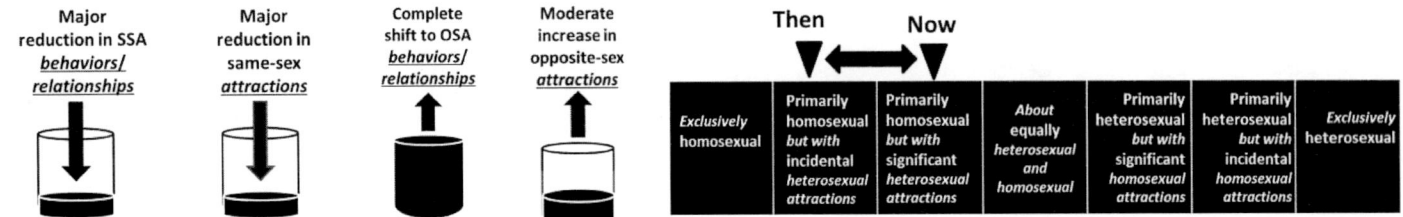

| **SSA "then"** | I "came out" as a gay man when I was 19 years old. I describe it as opening up the book of men, and closing, very firmly, the book of women. I believed that I was gay, and I accepted that as being my innate identity. For five years I lived with another man, and we had a very active homosexual sex life. |
|---|---|
| **Motivations** | I wanted to get married to a woman and to live according to my biological sexuality. |
| **SSA now** | Today, SSA is insignificant in my day-to-day life. I have been married to a woman for 25 years, and we have very enjoyable sex. |
| **What brought about change?** | Therapy, including a very important surrogate experience. I very much relate to the 12 Step system as being equally valid for my (and many others') SSA. The realization that my SSA is in essence an expression of an inner feeling that I lack masculinity. It comes exclusively from that place of not feeling man enough. |
| **Most helpful?** | My belief that heterosexuality is right, is what God wants, and is something I am capable of. |
| **Less helpful, or even harmful?** | I have not experienced, personally or from others, any harm that derived from these efforts. |
| **Any other benefits?** | I am much more able to help others, in sexuality-related issues and in empowerment issues. My sense of my own self-worth is much larger, as is my firm belief in my own healthy, heterosexual masculinity. |

# "James," 30, lives in Canada, Heterosexually Married, Christian

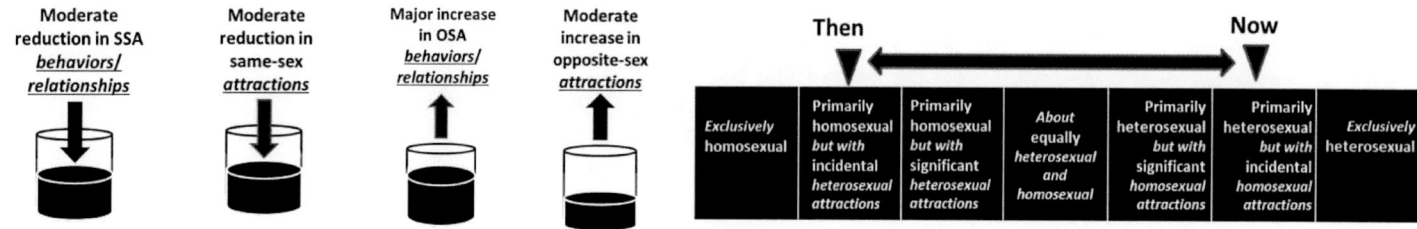

**Moderate reduction in SSA** *behaviors/ relationships*

**Moderate reduction in same-sex** *attractions*

**Major increase in OSA** *behaviors/ relationships*

**Moderate increase in opposite-sex** *attractions*

**Then** ◄─────────► **Now**

| *Exclusively homosexual* | **Primarily homosexual** *but with incidental heterosexual attractions* | **Primarily homosexual** *but with significant heterosexual attractions* | **About equally** *heterosexual and homosexual* | **Primarily heterosexual** *but with significant homosexual attractions* | **Primarily heterosexual** *but with incidental homosexual attractions* | *Exclusively heterosexual* |

**SSA "then"**

As a teenager, I was heavily addicted to pornography and meeting men online for sexual chat, etc. I would even come home during breaks at school to look at pornography and chat. I have not had sex with another man but definitely lived a double life. I was terrified of people finding out about my issue with same-sex attraction and was very lonely and miserable at that point in my life. I felt no attraction to women other than feeling like they were good friends. I liked hanging out with them and talking with them. I felt very alienated from other men in my life and my peers at school. I didn't feel like I was one of the guys, tried to connect with guys sexually via the Internet. I was very addicted and hated that part of myself. I felt no one understood.

**Motivations**

I have always wanted a traditional family to have kids of my own. Even though I was attracted to men, what I wanted was to have a wife and kids. I also hold very dearly to my heart religious beliefs that do not line up with living a gay lifestyle. To pursue a gay life would be to go against what I want and I what I believe.

**SSA now**

My same-sex attraction has decreased over time. Where I was once heavily addicted to pornography, it has now become a very occasional thing in my life. I feel much more the same as my peers and other men in my life. I am not attracted to men the way I was before, where I would feel this intense pull towards them. The same-sex attraction has decreased to the point where what I want most now is just close friendship with other men. I don't want to live with a man; I don't want a boyfriend. I still have not had sex with a man.

I have never been attracted to women in general, but in dating and falling in love with my wife, coupled with counseling, I can say I am very attracted to my wife and have very fulfilling, easy and enjoyable intimacy with her on a consistent basis. I desire her physically, sexually and romantically, which I never thought would have been possible 10 years ago. We have a great relationship. She knows all about my same-sex attraction, and our sex life is great. I more and more feel like women are "other," so I see them in a different way. I can say that my attraction for women has grown and continues to grow. Counseling and experiential weekends have played a major role in this.

**What brought about change?**

1) Went to counseling specifically around same-sex attraction issues prior to marriage.

2) Shared my struggles with my family and a few close friends. Shared with my wife prior to marriage.

3) Cut off some friendships that were unhealthy for me (unhealthy attachment to them or they had wrong intentions).

4) Put in place some accountability software around computers or anything with access to pornography.

5) Went on two intense experiential weekends focused around emotional healing related to SSA, which helped me work through some pain from my past and allowed me to go deeper with me in a safe way. It really helped me to feel like I wasn't alone and that I was one of the guys. I came

home changed, with much more peace and confidence in myself. My opposite sex- attractions grew the most as a result of these weekends.

**Most helpful?** Knowing there are other people who also have same-sex attraction but don't want to live it out was so helpful for me. It was nice to be with other men who also deal with this issue. The experiential weekends have really provided me a safe place to work through my pain and struggles with other men who understand. I have gotten a lot of freedom and confidence through these experiential weekends and the psychodrama that was part of it. I tell my wife that life makes the most sense to me when I am on an experiential weekend.

**Less helpful, or even harmful?** The most harmful thing for me is someone telling me that I have to live a gay life because I am attracted to men. I have never wanted that for me, don't believe it is right for me, and what I want I am living out right now. I am married to an amazing woman I love and have beautiful kids. I have the right to choose what life I want to live—and a gay life is NOT what I want or what is right for me. It is so harmful and hurtful to me to be told that what I am living is not right or that I am not being my true self.

**Any other benefits?** Yes, I have experienced a big change in my confidence and a large reduction in my anxiety— social anxiety and anxiety around other men. I feel much more comfortable around all types of men and have almost no anxiety, where those interactions were highly anxious for me before. I feel like a man more than I ever have before, I feel like one of the guys. I feel confident around women and feel very different from them. I definitely have greater self-esteem. I relate to my wife much better. I feel stronger internally and feel powerful to be able to do what I need to do in the world. I am a better dad and husband because of my sexual-orientation change efforts.

**Final comment?** I was at a point of despair before going to counseling as a young adult. I wanted to die and hated myself and where things were going. These change efforts were a lifeline to me that gave me hope, meaning, purpose, and helped me to live the life I want to live. My kids would not be here without these change efforts. I am so thankful for the people who are willing to help guys like me to live the life they want to live freely and with confidence.

# Tomasz, 44, lives in Poland, Single, Catholic

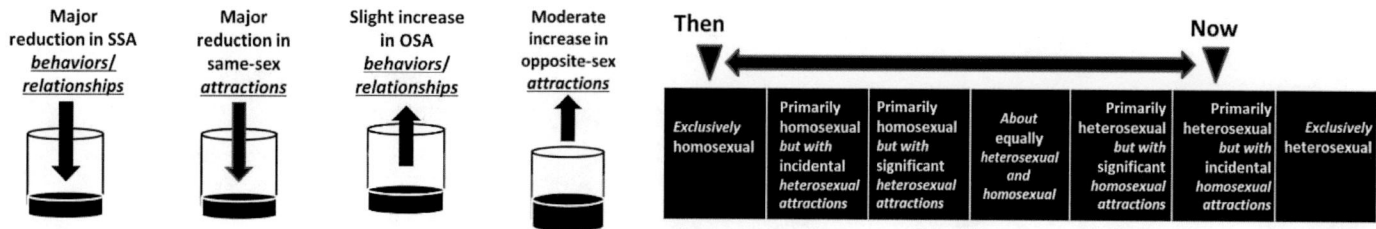

**SSA "then"**

I started to discover my SSA when I was about 12 to 14 years old. I observed it increasing, but hoped the SSA would disappear. When I was about 19 to 20 years old, I realized that those feelings will not disappear without any efforts. So I decided to do whatever possible to overcome it.

**Motivations**

My motivations were my Catholic religion and my relation with God. Also, fear of telling the truth about the homosexual feelings I experienced, and a desire to have my own family.

**SSA now**

My SSA is weak or even very week today. I am not sexually active.

**What brought about change**

- Psychotherapy (individual and group)
- Journey Into Manhood
- Noble Man
- New Warrior Training Adventure (NWTA)
- Religious retreats
- Developing my relationship with God
- Surrender prayer

**Most helpful**

My opinion about what was the most helpful has changed through the years. Very important was group psychotherapy for men with SSA. It was a new beginning for me. It allowed me to re-start my emotional life, which for unknown reasons apparently stopped at just a few years old.

Then Journey Into Manhood was very important, as well as Noble Man.

Finally however, I can say that Jesus Christ is the best psychotherapist. Therefore, currently I am focused on this aspect of my life. As of today, I see SSA as a defensive mechanism, to cope with fear in my life. God's love displaces that fear.

**Less helpful, or even harmful**

I have been a bit disappointed with NWTA, maybe because of high expectations. However, I can't say it was not helpful.

I have NEVER experienced any negative effects from any SSA change efforts. For me it is just the opposite. I WOULD experience negative effects if I had done nothing. That's my opinion.

**Other benefits?**

Definitely. All these efforts have given me incredible personal development in all aspects of my life.

## "Jerry," 43, lives in Maryland USA, Heterosexually Married, Jehovah's Witness

| Major reduction in SSA *behaviors/relationships* | Major reduction in same-sex *attractions* | No change in OSA *behaviors/relationships* (already satisfactory) | No change in opposite-sex *attractions* (already satisfactory) |
|---|---|---|---|

**Then** ◄──────────────────────► **Now**

| *Exclusively homosexual* | Primarily homosexual *but with* incidental heterosexual attractions | Primarily homosexual *but with* significant heterosexual attractions | *About equally heterosexual and homosexual* | Primarily heterosexual *but with* significant homosexual attractions | Primarily heterosexual *but with* incidental homosexual attractions | *Exclusively heterosexual* |
|---|---|---|---|---|---|---|

**SSA "then"**

There was a time when my same-sex attraction seemed to consume me. Though still attracted to my wife, I had this intense conflict going on inside, and I didn't know what to do. I started to go to places to meet men, such as gay bars and online gay dating services. I thought about leaving my wife because I must be gay. I still loved my wife and was still attracted to women, but I was consumed with attraction to men and I was miserable. I even thought at one point that suicide was an option. I just wanted these homosexual feelings to go away, but over time they seemed to just get worse.

**Motivations**

I was motivated by the fact that others I have heard of and spoken to have reduced or eliminated their homosexual attractions. What I have observed is that society offers people like me two choices: either you are gay and proud, or gay, closeted, and secretly wanting to come out. I was not happy with the conflict within myself, nor with the choices that society presented. I thought to myself, if others have reduced or eliminated their same-sex attraction, then this was something I wanted to investigate for myself.

**SSA now**

My SSA has been greatly reduced. There are days when it seems non-existent. I have noticed that when my SSA is reduced, my opposite-sex attractions naturally increase. I do not have urges to go to gay bars or try to have sex with men, and I do not want to leave my wife. Also, we enjoy a healthy, regular sex life.

**What brought about change?**

The weekend with People Can Change has been crucial for me in reducing my same-sex attraction. People Can Change has provided me with the tools I needed which have resulted in my experiencing a significant reduction and at times elimination of SSA. I have been working with a therapist in helping me heal my deep wounds that led to my SSA as well as working the Sexaholics Anonymous 12 Step program.

**Most helpful?**

Understanding what is behind same-sex attraction. I've come to realize that this attraction is an emotional one. When my core emotional needs are met by men in healthy ways, my SSA automatically decreases. The Journey Into Manhood weekend by People Can Change has helped me learn so much about myself and has taught me what I need to do to heal.

**Less helpful, or even harmful?**

Nothing. Everything that I learned through People Can Change, my therapist, etc., has been invaluable.

**Any other benefits?**

Yes. I have had a boost in self-confidence, in feeling more masculine and in knowing better how to form healthy relationships with men.

**Final comment?**

I can honestly say that the Journey Into Manhood weekend has helped me save my marriage and even my life. It has put me on a path of healing. My entire experience has been a positive one. I no longer feel despair like before. I no longer think of suicide as an option. I know I would not be happy living a gay life. Although the journey of healing has not been an easy one, it has been the best decision for me. I am happier, more confident, and enjoying life more now than ever before.

# Steve, 55, lives in Florida USA, Heterosexually Married, Jewish

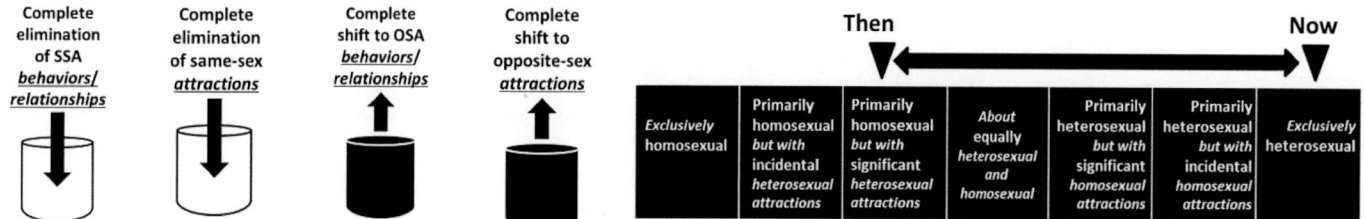

**SSA "then"**

Before I started this journey, I would "act out" with men secretly. These encounters were mostly in public and anonymous, with men I had never met before. I never even knew their names. Nevertheless, I did not identify as being gay. All of my family and friends viewed me as straight. In fact, I viewed myself as straight.

Over time, the amount of "acting out" increased, and at times this behavior would become obsessive and compulsive. I was very disturbed by this and had difficulty functioning as a result. I was sad, depressed and had difficulty sleeping. I felt shame and guilt. I wanted to stop, but couldn't.

**Motivations**

While I have had physical attraction to men, I never wanted any emotional connection with them. I never felt comfortable with my same-sex attractions. They resulted in shame and guilt. From an early age, I felt that I lacked something within. I would try to get this from sexual fantasy about men who, in my mind, had what I didn't. Later, this led to sexualization and loveless anonymous sexual encounters.

At the same time, I was drawn to loving and intimate relationships with women. I fell in love and got married, thinking that this could reduce the same-sex attractions. This did not work as I had intended. I set out to better understand my unwanted same-sex attraction.

Originally, I found an experiential therapy workshop that offered me significant benefit. I was able to understand the dynamic of my youth that led to my unwanted same-sex attraction. I had several years of complete heterosexuality without ANY same-sex attraction or fantasy. Only when my wife became very ill and was unable to support me any longer did my issue begin to resurface.

That is when I discovered the People Can Change community. Through their Journey Into Manhood, weekend, Journey Beyond and support groups, I was able to regain the path that I had previously taken. Without the weekends and the processes that they offer, I would not be the heterosexual man I am today.

**SSA now**

Through the work that I have done, the realizations of how childhood traumas affected me, and support for and from other men, I have been able to reverse the sexual behaviors of my past. I no longer "act out" with men (18 years), very rarely fantasize (six years), and I have a good, healthy attraction to women. I am aroused by women and have a healthy intimate relationship with my wife.

**What brought about change?**

In addition to experiential therapy and work within the People Can Change community, I have also used personal therapy, Sex Addicts Anonymous meetings and the ManKind Project to help maintain the success that I have achieved over the years.

**Most helpful?**

It is hard to say what was most beneficial to me. I believe that it was the work that I did in combination with the loving support of my wife.

| | |
|---|---|
| **Less helpful, or even harmful?** | Acting out sexually. Also, one therapist I saw told me that I was gay and that I should come out of the closet. I was offended and never went back to see him again. If only I could tell him how wrong he was. |
| | There have been no harmful effects from my efforts. In fact, it is only the opposite that has occurred. I was depressed and suicidal before this work. |
| **Any other benefits?** | I have had huge benefits unrelated to my unwanted SSA. I have become a man with self-esteem, integrity, and confidence. I am able to be a better husband, father, son, employer and human being. I understand my masculinity and am able to express it. I have honest, open and meaningful friendships that are based on who and what I truly am. I am happy and I help bring joy to those around me. This is not at all who I was before this work. |
| **Final comment?** | I have experienced dramatic change in sexual orientation/attraction. It is easy for someone to say this is impossible if they have not achieved it. |
| | I can't imagine where I would be today without this work. I don't think that I would be married. I might not even be alive. |

**C.D.,** 41, lives in Massachusetts USA, Heterosexually Married, Catholic

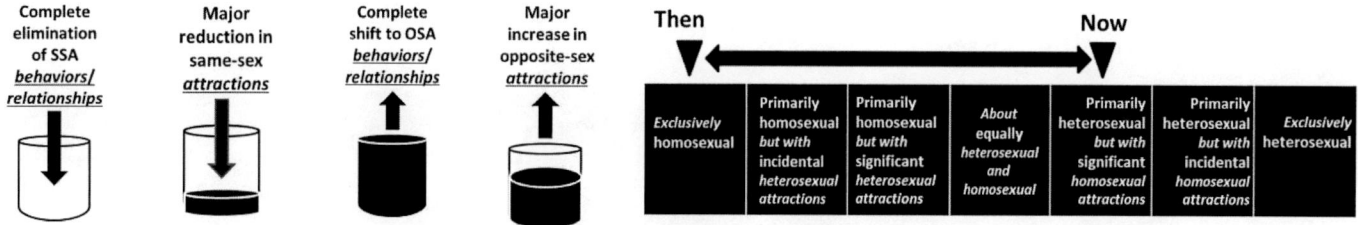

| | |
|---|---|
| **SSA "then"** | Everyone in the gay movement told me I had no choices—I was born that way, and the only options I had were to embrace the gay culture and the beliefs it promotes or enter into a suicidal and harmful exercise in self-denial. |
| **Motivations** | I reached a point in my life where the gay culture, gay movement and gay identity simply didn't fit me anymore. I no longer believed in the things that were important in the gay world. Furthermore, I had pretty much gotten "burned out" on gay sexuality and it really didn't turn me on the way it did when I first realized that not everyone was attracted to the same sex. |
| **SSA now** | Ultimately I decided to finally make my own decision and ignore the scare tactics I was getting from my gay friends and from the larger "movement." I defected from the gay culture because I didn't believe in it anymore. I discovered that I was capable of many different types of feelings, relationships and experiences that my gay-advocating friends had said weren't possible. I also learned that I wasn't the only person who experienced this type of change and that I was okay. I wish the gay apologists would quit their embittered quest to exterminate anyone who contradicts their ideas about victimization and immutability when it comes to sexual orientation. I hope more people get involved in People Can Change and have similar experiences to mine. |
| **What brought about change?** | Counseling, life coaching, SSA ministries, People Can Change, 12 Step group, experiential personal-growth weekends. |
| **Most helpful?** | If it hadn't been for People Can Change and reparative therapy, I don't know if I would have had the will to go on living in the gay culture and the disempowering beliefs it promotes. Seven years in, I am so glad I trusted it, so glad it works. |
| **Less helpful, or even harmful?** | Gay-affirming therapy was extremely harmful and disempowering. The entire process of pro-gay therapy (as I experienced it in groups and in church settings) was designed to reduce "who I was" to a very small and convenient sexual identity and then to blame all of my life's problems and unresolved feelings on society's unwillingness to accept that "type." |
| | If anything, it's gay-affirming therapy that should be outlawed because of the harm it does to people. I know some people who even contemplated suicide because gay-affirming groups, movements and therapists convinced them they had no power of discernment over their sexual orientation and could make no choices about how they would feel, live or form relationships if such choices even questioned "gayness" in any way. I found gay-affirming therapy to be extremely fraudulent and misleading because it promised a fulfillment, wholeness and peace that never came. |

# Rich, 53, lives in Virginia USA, Heterosexually Married, Latter-day Saint

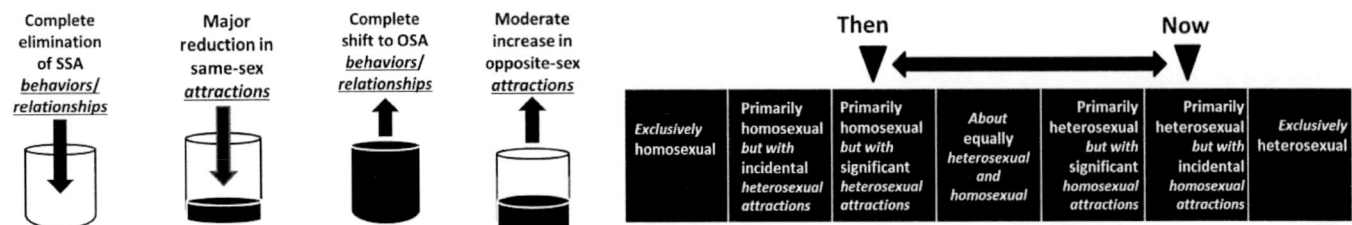

**SSA "then"**

Unlike most SSA men, my first sexual feelings in early puberty were for girls. But I also had the classic pre-homosexual home life (controlling, shaming mother; kind but distant father; strong bonds with sisters but no meaningful bonds with brothers). So I was at a tipping point to experience SSA when I began feeling bullied and alienated from boys at school, and at about the same time discovered gay pornography. I longed for male acceptance and belonging, and porn helped turn that natural longing into lust, then addiction. When I visited places that sold porn, men sought me out and gave me attention and (momentary) affection. I was hooked, but horribly conflicted.

After college, I briefly adopted a gay identity and lived a predominantly gay life for six months to a year. Then I discovered Sexaholics Anonymous and thought that was the answer. With my addiction temporarily under control, I fell in love with a woman, Marie, and we soon married. But because I hadn't resolved my underlying longings for healthy male connection, my addictive sexual patterns soon returned. I "acted out" with men, mostly anonymously, and lived a double life for nine years of my marriage. At the most hopeless point, I began to imagine suicide scenarios as a solution. Then I found reparative therapy and life-saving help.

**Motivations**

At one point, I was willing to walk away from my lifelong religion, reject my family of origin, and embrace a gay life if that's what it would take to bring peace. But the gay world (or at least gay Los Angeles in the late 1980s) greatly disappointed me. I found in it an obsession with sex, porn, youth and physical appearance; prevalent recreational drug use; a campy, effeminate "crush" on masculinity; and a derision of family life, monogamy and religion. I didn't like the man I became when I was with gay boyfriends or at their parties. In contrast, when I met Marie, I felt uplifted, like I was being called to be a better man. I liked the man I saw reflected in her eyes. That's who I really wanted to be.

**SSA now**

It has now been 18 years since I had any type of sexual connection with another man, and almost that long since I've even wanted to. I got sexually sober in 1997, and was completely faithful to my wife Marie for the second half of our marriage. Tragically, she died of cancer in 2006, but after her death I never once felt drawn to return to my former gay life or to hook up with men again. When I dated and remarried in 2010, it was wonderful to feel nearly 100% heterosexual, with none of the internal sexual conflict and confusion I had experienced when I was dating Marie in the late 1980s. I am very much in love again and completely attracted to my wife Janet, on every level. We have a very satisfying sex life. Most importantly, perhaps—I am at peace.

**What brought about change?**

I found a book, Born That Way?, that introduced me to the idea that change was actually possible. It led me to an SSA ministry, which led me to reparative therapy at Joseph Nicolosi's clinic in Los Angeles. (Read my personal experience with reparative therapy here.) Reparative therapy changed my whole world. I learned I had underlying needs for healthy male connection, and without meeting those natural, healthy needs I would seek out male connection sexually. I learned to embrace my own masculinity—something I hadn't realized I had never really done, due to a subconscious love-hate-fear of it. I worked a 12 Step program again, and got sexually sober. I became "initiated" into healthy masculinity through the New Warrior Training Adventure, and built deeply authentic male friendships. And I established two relationships with mentors who loved, accepted and supported me.

| **Most helpful?** | Reparative therapy; the New Warrior Training Adventure and follow-up groups; trusted, caring mentors; deep connections with new, trusted friends; getting sexually sober through Sexaholics Anonymous; and the support of a loving wife. All of this was guided by a deep spiritual connection and a humble submission to God's will for my life. |
|---|---|
| **Less helpful, or even harmful?** | The hate emails, phone calls or lies in online articles from people who don't know me but blame and attack me for walking away from a gay life, or for speaking out about my experience (and thus committing the "sin" of "blasphemy" against the approved, politically correct "gay talking points"). It's tragic that in order to speak my truth, and shine a beacon of light to others who might benefit, I and others have to be prepared to be publicly attacked and slandered. I welcome mutually respectful, civil dialogue that seeks to build mutual understanding on this issue and recognizes each individual's innate right to choose his own life path. Sadly, it seems that so few people have the capacity to really listen and respect different choices and beliefs. |
| **Any other benefits?** | With years of hindsight, I see that my SSA journey has become one of the great blessings of my life. I have more and deeper friendships than ever before. I am more emotionally balanced and grounded. I am free of lustful longings or addictive, out-of-control behaviors. I am a better husband, father and friend. I feel whole. I am at peace with who I am. |

# Section Seven:

# Questions and Answers

**Q. Hasn't scientific evidence proven that <u>reparative therapy</u> or other sexual-orientation change efforts (SOCE) don't work?**

A. No.

The idea that these efforts are ineffective is a political position taken by at least 13 large, mainstream U.S. mental health associations.[12] This position is **not** an unbiased conclusion drawn from scientific evidence. (How could it be? How can you prove a negative—that therapeutic interventions can never lead to sexual-orientation change for anyone?)

These trade groups or professional membership groups (that's what they really are, not unbiased scientific bodies) typically base their political positions on popular vote of their respective committees on gay and lesbian concerns—which are filled, invariably, by "out and proud" gays and lesbians.

But what does behavioral-science research *really* say?

Two very different professional organizations have done the most comprehensive review of the question of whether behavior-science research conducted over decades supports the idea that sexual orientation can change through therapy or other interventions, and have come to very different conclusions.

First, the American Psychological Association assembled a six-person task force in 2007 and tasked them to review all the research it could find on sexual-orientation change therapies, then determine whether the evidence indicated such therapies were effective. The outcome was pretty much pre-determined from the start—every one of the task force members was gay, a gay activist, or both. No therapists or researchers who actually worked in <u>reparative therapy</u> were allowed on the task force (although five highly qualified Ph.D. specialists in the field were recommended to the APA by the National Association for Research and Therapy of Homosexuality).[13] Any guesses how this turned out?

The APA task force came out in 2009 with its "<u>Report…on Appropriate Therapeutic Responses to Sexual Orientation</u>."[14] It reported that it had reviewed 83 studies published in English from 1960 to 2007. This in itself was a remarkable admission. The APA had previously claimed in its online newsroom that no such evidence existed at all, and here the task force found 83 such studies.[15]

The task force's conclusions? "Efforts to change sexual orientation are unlikely to be successful," "enduring change to an individual's sexual orientation is uncommon," reports of change could not be "empirically validated," and "compelling evidence" of change was "rare."

---

[12] <u>Just the Facts About Sexual Orientation and Youth: A Primer for Principals, Educators, and School Personnel</u>, 2008
[13]   <u>http://josephnicolosi.com/apa-task-force/</u>
[14]   <u>http://www.apa.org/pi/lgbt/resources/therapeutic-response.pdf</u>
[15] The National Association of Social Workers also falsely claimed that <u>"No data demonstrate that reparative or conversion therapies are effective…"</u> and the American Psych*iatric* Association continues to claim even today that <u>"There is no published scientific evidence supporting the efficacy of reparative therapy as a treatment to change one's sexual orientation."</u>

In summary, the all-gay task force concluded "there is insufficient evidence to support the use of psychological interventions to change sexual orientation" and "There are no studies of adequate scientific rigor to conclude _whether or not_ recent SOCE _do or do not work_ to change a person's sexual orientation" (emphasis added).

Sounds like a relatively neutral position, doesn't it? They reviewed 83 research studies and concluded: We're not convinced. It might or might not work.

And who decides what constitutes "adequate scientific rigor" anyway? Why, the task force, of course.

"Insufficient evidence" is a long way from claiming "no evidence." It's even further from proving the opposite—that these therapies have supposedly been proven to _not_ work. And yet that is what so many bloggers, "talking heads" and reporters have claimed the APA has said. (Remember: "…if you repeat [a lie] frequently enough, people will sooner or later believe it."[16])

A second professional organization—the much smaller, much more conservative National Association of Research and Therapy of Homosexuality—reviewed 600 reports of clinicians, researchers and former clients published over 125 years and published a comprehensive summary called "What Research Shows." NARTH is an advocacy group for therapists and researchers who support sexual-orientation change efforts. So, not surprisingly, it came to quite a different conclusion than the all-gay APA task force: There is in fact _substantial_ evidence that sexual orientation may sometimes be changed through reorientation therapies or related change efforts, the report said.

To learn more:

- A Formal Response to the Report of the American Psychological Association Task Force on Appropriate Therapeutic Responses to Sexual Orientation, by NARTH.

- APA Task Force—A Mockery of Science, by Joseph Nicolosi, Ph.D.

- Protect Client and Therapist Freedom of Choice Regarding Sexual Orientation Change Efforts, by Family Research Council.

- Can Sexual Orientation Change? (Chapter 12 from My Genes Made Me Do It! By Neil Whitehead, Ph.D., and Briar Whitehead).

- Why Science Doesn't Support Orientation-Change Bans, by Peter Sprigg.

## Q. Haven't sexual-orientation change efforts been proven to be harmful?

A. No.

There are anecdotes of perceived harm, certainly. But that experience is far from universal. And such "harm" could be in many cases as minimal as hurt feelings or a sense of wasted effort or regret—everyday human experience.

All the APA task force found in their review of 83 studies was that "some individuals perceived that they had benefited from SOCE while others perceived that they had been harmed." (Wouldn't that be true in every form of therapy or counseling on the planet?) And: "We cannot conclude how likely it is that harm will occur from SOCE."[17] As Peter Sprigg of the Family Research Council has written, "The (APA's) statement that SOCE 'may' cause distress

---

[16] Psychoanalyst Walter Langer
[17] http://www.apa.org/pi/lgbt/resources/therapeutic-response.pdf

(not 'has caused,' 'will cause,' or 'often causes') is about as weak as it could possibly be—amounting to little more than speculation."[18]

Notice how psychologists, gay activists and others who reject first-hand accounts of successful change efforts based on the fact that those accounts are just anecdotes, not quantitative research, are so quick to embrace and trumpet any anecdotal reports of harm as representative of sexual-orientation interventions generally.

As we've seen, many of us who have been profiled in this book experienced significant harm *before* seeking out change therapies or other change programs—up to and including suicidal thoughts or even suicide attempts (see Section Five, "Any Harm?" page 35). That is, until we found hope for minimizing our unwanted same-sex attractions, eliminating unwanted behaviors, and distancing our sense of self from homosexual feelings.

Many of us also experienced great frustration, shame and a sense of personal boundary violations when therapists or others told us we could not change and we had no choice but to accept an identify and lifestyle we did not want. (see Section Five, "Any Harm?" page 32). Is no one concerned about the harm that can befall *us*?

As anyone can see from this book, there is a significant group of people who have benefited greatly from our sexual-orientation change efforts. In many cases, those efforts even saved our lives.

## Q. What really happens in <u>reparative therapy</u>?

A. Reparative therapy (or other forms of sexual-orientation change therapies) has been falsely caricatured online and in the media. But at its essence, reparative therapy is basically talk therapy, using the same techniques that therapists use for all kinds of unwanted behaviors or emotional pain. This type of therapy and these types of change efforts are about building self-esteem, affirming one's right to choose one's own life path, and uncovering and healing underlying emotional pain. They are about releasing shame, affirming a man's innate masculinity, and helping him connect more easily with other men around him.

Sometimes people who know nothing about these therapy programs describe aversion techniques that haven't been used for 50 years or more, and pretend that those are representative of modern therapeutic techniques. Sometimes opponents have made up alleged abuse stories altogether. Like the male-to-female transgendered person who testified before the New Jersey legislature that as a child she had been subject to torturous shock therapy at a particular "gay conversion camp" in Ohio called True Directions. But fact checkers found no evidence that any such camp existed—except in a 1999 movie called *But I'm a Cheerleader.*[19] Or alleged abuse survivor Sam Brinton, who, oddly enough, can't seem to recall the name of the therapist who supposedly tortured him, so his story can't be fact checked.[20]

Please, disregard the manufactured claims, archaic practices and cartoonish portrayals. Listen to us who have experienced reparative therapy and other sexual-orientation change efforts for ourselves. We found them respectful, appropriate, effective, and ultimately life-changing, for the better.

To learn more:

- <u>What is Reparative Therapy? Examining the Controversy</u>, by Joseph Nicolosi, Ph.D.

- <u>A Change of Heart: My Two Years in Reparative Therapy</u>, by Rich Wyler

[18]    http://www.firstthings.com/web-exclusives/2013/09/why-science-doesnt-support-orientation-change-bans
[19]    http://www.wnd.com/2013/03/transgendered-woman-lies-about-therapy-torture/, http://www.njfpc.org/nj-reparative-therapy-ban-us-court/, http://townhall.com/columnists/michaelbrown/2013/03/25/did-a-gay-activist-lie-to-the-new-jersey-senate-n1548304/page/full
[20]    http://www.christianpost.com/news/ex-gay-therapy-debate-the-truth-matters-125479/, http://www.frcblog.com/2014/08/truth-matters-ex-gay-debate/

## Q. What if I want to work on diminishing my same-sex attractions. Where do I start?

A. To begin with, make sure that you are intrinsically motivated to pursue change, in order to be true to yourself and your own life goals and beliefs. Never pursue change just to try to make other people happy. If you are man who is committed to pursuing change, we recommend you pursue a path in which you regularly ask yourself:

What changes can I make in the way I'm thinking and the things I'm doing with my life that can help me to:

- Like and accept myself more

- Better connect to my own masculinity in non-sexual ways

- Build a network of supportive brothers with whom I can build lasting, authentic, non-sexual relationships

- Uncover and heal underlying emotional pain

- Discover and meet underlying, core needs

- Surrender or release shame, harmful thoughts and destructive behaviors, and anything that is blocking me from being the man I want to be, or that I feel called to be.

This program is summarized in the "M.A.N.S." acronym developed for the Journey Into Manhood program. In fact, reading that summary is a good place to start your journey. Here are some other steps to get started:

1. **Begin by simply reading and learning.**

   - See a comprehensive book list on the People Can Change website.

   - And spend some time reading the website itself, especially the section, "Our Solution: A M.A.N.S. Journey."

2. **Look into support groups or online discussion groups.**

   - "Journey Together," People Can Change's professionally facilitated life-coaching group

   - Worldwide peer-led video groups by Joel225

   - People Can Change's Yahoo- and Facebook-based discussion and support groups

   - Online support through Courage, especially for Catholics

   - Email discussion groups, especially for Mormons

   - Email discussion groups, especially for Jews

3. **Next, find a therapist or life coach.**

   - There is a short list on the People Can Change website of counselors and life coaches who have first-hand knowledge of People Can Change and its programs.

   - Or find a therapist through NARTH by making an online referral request.

4. **If your sexual behaviors are out of control, compulsive or addictive, look into a sexual addiction recovery program:**

- Sexaholics Anonymous (also check into its phone- and Internet-based groups)

- Sex Addicts Anonymous (also check into its phone- and Internet-based groups)

- Celebrate Recovery.

5. **Also, look into the experiential-healing and personal-growth programs that so many other men have found helpful—or even life-changing:**

- Journey Into Manhood

- Adventure In Manhood

- Noble Man

- Edge Venture

- New Warrior Training Adventure (but see cautions about this program to make sure it is right for you)

In all of this, remember:

- Take charge of your own destiny. Don't let anyone else tell you who you are, or what you should feel, or what path is appropriate for you.

- Know that you are good and valuable just as you are—right now, today, unchanged, and even if you never change. Never allow shame to drive your life choices. Never allow shame to define you.

- Remember that the ultimate goal isn't heterosexuality—it is peace. Oftentimes heterosexuality emerges or increases almost as a byproduct of doing this work—but there are no guarantees. And besides, heterosexuality alone can never promise happiness.

- Have realistic expectations (see "How Much Change?" page 19). Don't expect too much change too fast. Accept yourself where you are. As they say in the 12 Step programs: "Progress, not perfection."

There is a reason we call this a journey.